IT'S NOT
ABOUT
THE HAIR

It's Not About the Hair
And Other Certainties of Life & Cancer

Debra Jarvis

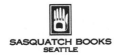

SASQUATCH BOOKS
SEATTLE

For Wes, my one and only.

These stories are true, but all names and identifying characteristics of patients have been changed to ensure confidentiality.

Printed in the United States of America
Published by Sasquatch Books

18 17 16 15 14   20 19 18 17 16 15 14 13 12

First paperback edition, 2008

Cover photograph: David Belisle
Cover design: Rosebud Eustace
Interior design and composition: Scott Taylor/FILTER/Talent

Library of Congress Cataloging-in-Publication Data

Jarvis, Debra.
        It's not about the hair : and other certainties of life and cancer / Debra Jarvis.
        p. cm.
ISBN-13: 978-1-57061-536-8/ISBN-10: 1-57061-536-5 (hardcover)
ISBN-13: 978-1-57061-573-3/ISBN-10: 1-57061-573-X (paperback)
        1. Jarvis, Debra—Health. 2. Breast—Cancer—Patients—Biography. 3. Breast—Cancer—Psychological aspects. I. Title.
RC280.B8.J32 2007
362.196'994490092—dc22
[B]
                                        2007013055

Sasquatch Books
1904 Third Avenue, Suite 710
Seattle, WA 98101
(206) 467-4300
www.sasquatchbooks.com
custserv@sasquatchbooks.com

CONTENTS

INTRODUCTION

I am the general oncology outpatient chaplain at the Seattle Cancer Care Alliance (SCCA). I see patients who are receiving chemotherapy, getting radiation, having their blood drawn, or waiting to see their oncologists. I was in my fourth year at the SCCA when I received the upsetting news that my mother had been diagnosed with breast cancer. However, I didn't have much time to be disturbed about it because five days later *I* was diagnosed with breast cancer. I couldn't decide if her case or mine was the most disturbing, so I settled on being equally disturbed about both.

Still, like having your car break down when you work at an auto repair shop, I thought if you had to have cancer, it was pretty convenient to work at a place that treats it.

"But you're the chaplain! You should be immune!" I heard this from a lot of outraged people, as if I had some special spiritual protection.

So what if I'm the chaplain? I'm a Christian, the faith that's all about the crucifixion of the guy who is considered the Son of God! I mean if the *Son of God* can't get a break, why should I? I'm only the chaplain.

So I chose to have my surgery and chemotherapy at the University of Washington, the medical center affiliated with SCCA. During my first appointment with my oncologist she made it clear she completely understood if I wanted to go elsewhere if I felt uncomfortable or for reasons of privacy.

"Why," I asked, "would I not want to be treated at a place that is filled with people I know and love? And why would I not want to be treated at a place where I have witnessed the finest care given in my twenty years as a hospital chaplain? And above all, why would I not want to be treated at a place where I know the location of every single restroom?"

She got my point.

Besides knowing the staff and the location of the restrooms, I had another advantage. I had seen people deal with cancer a thousand different ways—some inspiring and some less so. I've listened to patients who tried to pretend cancer is a million yuks. It's not. It's not even a hundred.

And I've listened to people who are whiny and tragic. Even if your situation *is* tragic, it doesn't feel good to whine—for very long. Forgive me if I sound harsh. I'm not talking about expressing your feelings, I'm talking about whining, and there is a difference.

Whining is basically about being stuck. You are stuck telling the same story in the same way in spite of everyone's efforts to help you resolve it or reframe it or find meaning in it.

Somewhere between the joking and whining, there is this precious place of absolute centeredness—peace in the eye of upheaval and chaos. It is an assertive kind of peace because it takes effort to stay grounded and centered while things swirl around you. It's not as if you're just sitting there blissed out, denying your pain or your fear. It means you feel your feelings, give them a voice, and then move on.

I read a new patient's chart and thought, "Holy-Jesus-God-and-All-the-Saints! What a disaster!" But then I met this patient, and she was all upbeat and grateful for this and grateful for that. She said, "Here's a funny thing that happened on my way to brain surgery . . ."

I wanted to say, "Have you read your chart lately?" But I could tell she knew exactly what was going on and was being completely authentic. It was all in how she chose to be with her situation. She was her Best Real Self.

That's how I wanted to be: my Best Real Self. For some people that means being more private about it, but for me, that meant being very open about my diagnosis. So I sent out e-mail updates on my treatment progress. Friends and family wanted information, and they also wanted to know *how I was* with what was going on. And my therapist friends wanted to know how I was with how I was.

Knowing that time is precious and e-mail can be overwhelming, I included just a few thoughts and feelings in each message. I wanted to write more about what surprised me, what helped me, and what disappointed me, but it didn't feel right to send six page e-mails. It's an e-mail, not an electronic book.

I learned much about cancer from being a patient, and probably the most astounding thing to discover was only a small part of the cancer experience is about medicine. Most of it is about feelings and faith, and losing and finding your identity, and discovering strength and flexibility you never knew you had. It's also about looking at life and staring death in the eye. It's about realizing the most valuable things in life are not things at all, but relationships. It's about laughing in the face of uncertainty and having the courage to ask for more chocolate and less broccoli.

And, if you haven't figured it out by now, it's about realizing cancer is *the best* excuse for getting out of practically anything— except chemotherapy.

And although many people asked me how I felt about it, what it was going to be like to lose it, and how I was going to deal with not having it . . . it's *not* about the hair.

One

A BIZARRE TWIST OF FATE

Dear Family and Friends,

Last Wednesday I was shocked and dismayed to find out my mother was diagnosed with breast cancer. It is Ductal Carcinoma In Situ (DCIS), and it is curable with a lumpectomy.

In a bizarre twist of fate, this past Tuesday *I* was diagnosed with breast cancer. Always competitive, my tumor is a teeny bit more serious: Stage I, infiltrating ductal carcinoma.

My first thought was, "Now I can be in the first wave at the Danskin Triathlon!"

My second thought was, "Oh, shit."

I tried to go back to that first thought, seeing myself in the group of cancer survivors who start the triathlon swim, but my mind kept going back to, "Oh, shit."

But the cancer is, in my friend/surgeon's words, "Curable!" In the past I thought of the word only in reference to hams and salami. I never thought I would be grateful to have it applied to me.

At first I thought we could take care of things with a lumpectomy. Well, I went from lumpectomy to mastectomy when DCIS was discovered in another quadrant of my breast. My surgeon looked very apologetic as he explained he couldn't just take a scoop out here and a scoop out there because, uh—well, there wasn't a lot of tissue to begin with and . . . uh . . .

"You mean," I said, "it would be like scooping ice cream. Two scoops from a gallon is no big deal, but two scoops from a pint—well, that leaves a mess so you might as well just eat the whole thing."

He nodded but looked vaguely nauseated by this comparison.

But now we had a plan, so I could call my parents and give them the news. It was just hideous telling them, although I tried to be really upbeat. My mom answered, and I'll tell you right now that my voice gets very high when I lie.

"Hi, Mom! Talk about coincidence! Can you believe it? I have breast cancer, too!" I sounded like a shrill game show host giving out the grand prize. She didn't buy it. I could tell by the strangling sound on the other end of the phone. It turns out her surgery is scheduled soon after mine—too soon for me to be with her for hers.

I'm not overjoyed to have cancer, but I do feel very cared for and held and safe. I'm not keeping this a secret, because I refuse to participate in the shame and stigma around cancer. I figure the more people who know, the more prayers and support! I have a friend whose husband has advanced prostate cancer, and he refuses to tell anyone. She is buckling under the strain.

My dear husband, Wes, is doing okay, although it took a while for it to really sink in. It was the session with my surgeon and all those words like "margins," "malignant," and "sentinel node," that made him know this was really happening.

One of my patients said, "Wow, having cancer will make you connect even more with your patients!"

I said, "If I connect any more with my patients I'll be having sex with them."

I would have liked to call each one of you, but I've had so many invitations to mammograms, ultrasounds, biopsies, and MRIs. My cancer dance card is full.

Anyway, there you have it. Thanks for all your support and prayers.

Love and Hugs,
Debra

Strength Training

The night before my breast biopsy I was emceeing a benefit concert for Multifaith Works, a Seattle agency for people with AIDS. It was the fourth year I had done this, and I loved getting all dressed up, introducing musical acts, and cracking jokes. It was basically being a diva for a night. That night I was wearing a teal blue jersey knit dress with cutaway armholes and a plunging neckline. It was not the kind of dress with which you could wear a bra. This didn't matter to me because I've never had huge boobs. I loved the way I felt in the dress—like a million bucks.

Before I left the house that night I looked closely at myself in the mirror, and I thought about the biopsy the next day. Like a lightning bug on a summer evening, the question flickered through my mind, "How long will I be able to wear this dress?" Then the thought was gone, and it was time for the show!

After the concert, a little boy came up to me and asked, "Are you strong?"

His mother laughed and said, "He's been looking at your arms all night."

"I've been training for a triathlon," I explained. "So I guess I am pretty strong."

The biopsy the next day was just tolerable. I wasn't screaming, but I was *so* wishing I wasn't lying there having my breast shot with a tiny spear gun. The "area of concern" was close to my chest wall and difficult for the doctor to reach. I noticed no one used the word "suspicious" probably because it makes patients feel, well—suspicious.

When the doctor was finally done, she bandaged me up and gave me this darling little ice pack to stick in my bra. It was round, about the size of a small biscuit. I saw immediately that once it was thawed, it could be used to, how shall I say—enhance the overall contours of the chest area. Marvelous. I asked for another one so I could have a matching pair.

Within five minutes of getting dressed, the local anesthetic wore off, and my breast was throbbing. I ran into one of my doctor buddies on the way out of the clinic.

"This is hurting way more than I thought," I said. "What should I take for the pain?"

"Do you have anything else to do today?"

"No."

"Take two Percocet."

"And call you in the morning?"

The two Percocet did the job with my pain. But the next morning, to my surprise, my breast had gone up a whole cup size!

"Looks like you had a bleed in there," Wes said.

He was right, but there was nothing to do now but wait. And wait.

I'm pretty good about stuff like this—I don't usually spend all day obsessing. So I went about my usual activities. But in the same way your tongue goes to a bite mark in your mouth, I would think, "Biopsy? What's going to happen with that?" I didn't stay there long though. I've spent hundreds of hours talking with people about how it's a waste of energy to worry about what you can't change. So a little of that sunk in.

Five days later I still hadn't received the results of my biopsy. I kept checking for my results online, which is a benefit of getting care at the medical facility in which you work. Many people were horrified about this, but I was insanely curious and knew I wouldn't freak out whatever the results were.

That morning I "accidentally" ran into a friend of ours who is a surgeon with the clinic. (Hereafter known as Our Friend The Surgeon.) He asked me what was new, and I told him about my mom and how I was waiting for my biopsy.

"Biopsy?" He called down to the pathology lab, but it wasn't ready, and he asked them to call him as soon as it was. He said he'd page me the second he knew.

Okay, here is what is totally bizarre about that encounter: I almost never see him in the clinic, let alone the south stairwell. The couple times I have seen him, he is crazy busy and as much as I love this guy, I wouldn't dream of asking him to stop and chat. How is it that I worked there three years and never saw him there before and have not yet seen him there again?

I was pretty busy seeing patients all day. That afternoon I said to myself, "Be a good dog and finish all your charting, and then you can look up your results." It was a beautiful day in April, and I was sitting in this gorgeous temporary office I had. The sun was streaming through the window, and I was a happy little clam sitting there writing charts. I finished. Good dog! Then I looked up my pathology report.

"Infiltrating ductal carcinoma, Nottingham grade I/III."

I had this immediate physiological reaction: instant sweat and pounding heart. The feeling was a lot like how you feel when you serendipitously spot someone on whom you have a major crush. But there was no ensuing fantasy. I got up to see if any of my doctor friends were around, but of course, they were seeing patients. I had this urge to tell somebody right away.

So I called Wes. He is a research scientist/physician and is always in the lab or in the clinic or in a meeting. He was actually at his desk—another minor miracle. I said, "Okay, so I have cancer. Here's what it said." Then I read him the report. He later told me he was shocked and afraid, and that he was standing but couldn't feel the bottoms of his feet. He also wanted to do something immediately. I guess he was a little upset.

He said, "Page Our Friend The Surgeon." So I did, and just as I was hanging up the phone, there was a knock at the door, and it was Our Friend The Surgeon!

He walked in and said, "Just a minute, I've got a page."

I said, "Don't worry. It's me!" Then he saw I was online. I said, "Yeah, so I read it. What does this mean?"

He looked at me and said, "Well, it's invasive cancer, but it's curable. I've got you scheduled for an MRI on Wednesday." I mean the guy was *on top of it!* That was so great. Then Wes called, and I put him on the phone with Our Friend.

While they talked I remembered the little boy at the concert asking me, "Are you strong?"

I guess I would find out.

Putting on the Ritz

I always tried to visit all the patients in the clinic who were receiving their first dose of chemotherapy. That first visit is overwhelming. You don't know where to park, where the elevators and restrooms are, how to register, or where the best seat in the waiting room is. You don't know your nurse, what chemo is going to feel like, or if you'll get any food. For this reason, when I make that first visit, I act sort of like a concierge at an upscale hotel.

I want to assure the patients we will do our best to care for them. I want them to see me, the chaplain, as a friend and servant, not some powerful authority to be feared. I mean "servant" in the sense of "one who serves," not in the sense of "slave."

People get wigged out over that word "serve," but I think it would be a different world if everyone thought about their job as a way to serve the world instead of a way to make money.

What would it be like if when your alarm went off you thought, "I've got to get up and go in to serve?" Or at a party, instead of asking, "So what do you do?" ask, "So how do you serve?" This doesn't mean you have to be in the Peace Corps, or adopt orphans, or run a homeless shelter. I think you can serve the world by being a joyful presence as you hand over that latte or make copies for your boss.

So on my first visit as concierge/chaplain I might say, "Hi, I'm Debra, the general oncology chaplain. I like to peek in and say hi to everybody on their first visit. Are you finding everything you need? How's the room service? Have they brought you any cookies?" This usually breaks the ice. They like that I'm not asking them anything medical or anything religious.

Then I usually ask, "So what brings you to our fine establishment today? I know it's not the lunches." I say this because it's funny, but the truth is I love the lunches. So then they tell me their stories.

The first few minutes are always a test. They want to know if I'm really interested, do I really care? Or am I going to sit there and nod and say, "Mm-hmm," like the stereotype of a Freudian shrink?

Jeff Spalding started with, "I was born in Spokane and there were eight kids in my family." I settled in, because often, if someone starts out with his birthplace, I know I'm there for a while. Jeff was about thirty-five, had a buzz cut, and looked like he spent his days not driving Peterbilt trucks, but lifting them over his head. It turned out that Jeff started with his birthplace because it was relevant to his current experience.

"So all my family still lives in Spokane, and I don't really have any family out here. One day I was lifting weights and I just passed out. And I thought I was dehydrated, so I drank some water and started lifting again and passed out again. So I went to my doctor. He ran some tests. Turned out I have esophageal cancer!"

"What?! That totally sucks."

"Yeah, I was floored."

My reaction usually matches their reaction even if I already know their diagnosis. This is because while they are telling me the story, I am right there with them. So I was right there with Jeff in the gym thinking he was dehydrated. And I was right there with him when his doctor said, "Esophageal cancer."

I reached over and squeezed his enormous bicep. "Yup," I said. "I can see that you are not exaggerating about this weight lifting thing." He gave me a big grin, and then I knew I had passed the test.

On that very first visit with Jeff, it was clear that his most important source of support was his family. I could tell by the way he said, "All my family still lives in Spokane." He had been diagnosed only a few weeks ago, and I knew he was still in that stage where you think you are watching a movie about cancer and you happen to be the star.

"I just don't know how I got this," he said. "I was taking supplements and stuff to build my muscles. Could it be that? I don't even have any cancer in my family. Maybe it was all those electrolyte drinks—and they didn't even taste that good!"

On the first visit I never press anyone to have a conversation about his or her spirituality. I just wait. I can do this because I have the luxury of seeing patients for the length of their chemo, which is often weekly or bi-monthly for at least a few months. There are only a couple of other clinics in the United States that have chaplains for outpatients. I think it's the best chaplain gig going because there is time to develop a relationship.

It's not like working in a hospital where the stay can be brief, or the emergency room, where all you get is one shot. It's the difference between a drive-through burger joint and a four-star restaurant. I'm not just handing you your food, I'm here to serve you and to have a relationship with you. You are a repeat customer. There is no rush. May I suggest the chicken noodle soup?

I mean this literally as well as metaphorically. Just before I leave the room I always ask, "Is there anything I can get for you? Would you like a bottle of water or some cookies?" Most people are surprised and delighted by this. The nurses and nursing assistants all do the same thing, and it helps a patient feel like a welcomed guest. Yeah, yeah, we all know you're in a cancer center, but why not make the experience for everyone as pleasant as possible? Looking at it in a totally selfish light, it just feels better to be thoughtful and kind rather than selfish and uncaring.

How Did I Cause It?

Although I am a graduate of the Shit Happens School of Cause and Effect, when I got my cancer diagnosis, I did exactly what Jeff did when he got his: I tried to figure out how I got it. I regularly exercise, am in a happy marriage, and eat well. But here are the things that immediately came into my mind:

Too many protein bars! That summer when low-carb was all the rage I ate chocolate/peanut butter protein bars all day long. I also ate those low-carb fake candy bars that contain artificial sweeteners such as acesulfame potassium and neotame. Frightening to pronounce let alone ingest.

Not enough meditation! I had a good meditation practice going for a while, but, well, things got busy—um, yeah. Maybe meditation would have calmed down any abnormal rapidly dividing cells. Or perhaps the Divine was trying to tell me something, but I wasn't there to listen.

I should tell you that I use these words interchangeably: God, the Divine, the Universe, the Presence, Mr. Martha Miyagi. I'll explain that last one. I don't have a visual for "God." She/He/It has always been an inner voice for me—a combination of Mr. Miyagi from *The Karate Kid*, and Martha Stewart—before she became a felon. I figured that Mr. Martha Miyagi said, "Well, cancer ought to slow her down. That will give her time to meditate." I got very zealous about meditating right then because I was afraid that if I didn't the Universe would cut off my legs.

Didn't take a real lunch! I had a bad habit of working through lunch. This was usually because a lot of patients came in between 11 a.m. and 2 p.m. If I took lunch then I'd miss them. Then in the late afternoon, I would eat lunch at my desk while charting. This is not considered good self-care. But I thought, "What if the patients who don't see me this week die?" It gradually dawned on me that if they did die, it would probably be because of their cancer, not because they didn't see me.

Fired from my job! Seven years before my diagnosis I had been fired for a book I wrote, and I was devastated—much weeping and gnashing of teeth! The stress of that must be what caused it.

So those are all the reasons my mind provided. But I know that I can never trust my mind. So I meditated and went deep within and asked my heart, "What caused my cancer?"

My heart said, "*Shit happens.*"

Moderate Dread

A few weeks before my diagnosis I read an interview with a psychologist who said, "Familiarity moderates dread." I think that is exactly right. If you told me I had multiple sclerosis I'd probably be so freaked out, I'd be chewing off my own arm. But cancer was something I knew. It would be surgery, chemo, radiation, hormonal therapy, or some combination of them.

Or maybe it was my twenty-plus years of working with the terminally ill and cancer patients that led me to think it was just a matter of time before I was diagnosed. Before my biopsy report came back a nurse friend asked me, "What is your intuition about this?"

I said, "There is something in there. It's not really bad, but it's something." So I wasn't shocked when my biopsy report came back stating cancer. I knew I wasn't going to die from it—at least not right away, and here's why.

One night when I was on-call, about a year before my diagnosis, I was asked to come in and talk with a family about withdrawing life support from their father. He was in the intensive care unit, had untreatable metastatic lung cancer, and had been comatose for weeks. He had made it clear to his children that he didn't want to linger on life support.

I was quite grouchy about this call since I had worked all day, and now I had to drive all the way back to the hospital. But I figured we'd talk, they'd withdraw support, and that would be that.

It turned out that his two sons didn't want to withdraw life support until the next morning. And they didn't need to talk about it, they just wanted to meet me and see if I was the right person to lead them in prayer before their father died. So actually, it was a job interview.

They were really wonderful men and before we left that night we prayed together. When we stood up to leave, the eldest put his hand on my arm. I looked up at him. He had the oddest look on his face.

He said, "Sometimes when I pray I see things." He hesitated for a moment and then said, "I just want you to know that there is still yet much work for you to do."

He said it with love, gentleness, and absolute certainty. We silently looked at one another for a moment. I did not feel afraid as if some fortune-teller predicted my future doom. Instead, I felt an overwhelming gratitude, as if I were running a race and someone was cheering me on with the words, "Hill ahead! Go for it, you'll be fine!"

I hugged him and thanked him. This happens all the time in ministry—you think you are going to help someone, and it turns out that they are there to help you. Sometimes they don't even know they're helping you, but this guy knew.

As I drove home that night I thought, "Something is coming that will cause a delay, but will not shut down my entire life." I felt calm, and well, curious. I also felt slightly embarrassed that I was so damn cranky about going to the hospital.

So when I found out I had cancer I thought, "Ah-ha! So *that's* the delay."

What's Your Story?

Patients have to know that I really care, that I'm not there to convert them or judge them or quiz them on their theology. I try to create a welcoming space for them to tell their stories without fear. If they can do this, then most people are able to reflect on their own pain and suffering, and hopefully are able to befriend and to find their truth in their stories.

What does this mean to befriend your story? Is this some kind of New Age crap or counselor speak? No. It means that you can tell the story of your past, with whatever pain or joy or grief it contains, and tell it without shame and with some insight about who you are today and who you might become.

Some people can hardly stand to think about from where they've come, let alone tell anyone else about it. Gabriela was one of these people. She was a beautiful seventy-five-year-old Puerto Rican lady. She reminded me of a short, stocky Elizabeth Taylor. Unlike Liz, Gabriela was very shy and quiet, and she was getting chemotherapy for colon cancer. She came in with her husband, and when I asked about her he answered for her in his big booming voice.

"She was born in Puerto Rico! Her dad was a fisherman." The louder he got the more she sunk into the bed and pulled the blankets around her until she looked like a tiny little speck of pepper on a mound of mashed potatoes. I tried talking with her about growing up there, but she didn't want to talk about it.

It was months before she told me that she hated for anyone to know she was from Puerto Rico because she moved to the States as a child, and all the kids made fun of the way she spoke. Because she was speaking flawless English, I almost didn't believe her, but I could hear the pain in her voice.

I also noticed that when one of the cleaning staff came in to empty the wastebaskets, Gabriela never greeted her, and once muttered under her breath, "Does she even speak English?"

Gabriela hated her own story, and for her to make friends with it, she would have to recognize that as a child she was the victim of prejudice and cruelty, and the children were wrong to make fun of her. But because she had never let go of her hurt and resentment, she didn't have any insight into her own behavior. She was still angry with some little kids who were mean to her back in the 1930s. So she became prejudiced and mean herself. But she just as easily could become compassionate and kind.

The next time the cleaning staff emptied the wastebaskets, I turned to Gabriela and said, "You have to admire her for learning English and finding a job. It's so scary to come to a foreign country." Gabriela didn't say a word, but I could tell she took that in.

Do I know if she became compassionate and kind? No. I'd like to say every pastoral encounter is like a Disney movie with a happy ending, but sometimes it's more like an indie film where everyone files out of the theatre saying, "Huh?"

But You're the Chaplain!

At least a dozen people said to me, "You? Cancer? But you're the chaplain!" And I found myself saying, "Well, why not?" It made me wonder if there were any occupations where a cancer diagnosis would be more acceptable. Meter maid? Dogcatcher? IRS agent?

It amused me that people thought a job in the ministry would somehow exempt me from any badness in my life. "The rain falls on the just and the unjust." It's a pisser, but it's true.

I must confess that in my prayer and meditation that question did come up. I asked, "So, yeah, what's up with the breast cancer?"

Ah, Grasshopper, that's for me to know and for you to find out.

"I hate it when you get all mysterious on me."

Trust me, it is a good thing.

That's the kind of stuff I hear from God. But that's my point really—that I do hear from the Divine. I never felt as if Mr. Martha Miyagi just hung up on me. And when I think back to the most painful times in my life, they all eventually led me somewhere better. So far I've had a resurrection for every time I've felt crucified. But it's taken *a lot* longer than three days.

At this point perhaps you are wondering about my take on Jesus. I *do* have a visual for Jesus because I grew up seeing pictures of him: the hair, the robe, the sandals, and the beard. If God the Father is Mr. Martha Miyagi to me, do I consider Jesus to be son of Mr. Martha Miyagi? In my mind, Jesus is closer to *Jon* Stewart than to Martha Stewart. I truly think he has a sense of humor, although my money is on her when it comes to fishes and loaves.

Whenever I read the Gospels, I get the distinct feeling that Jesus was really kind of a wise-ass, but that the Gospel writers cut out all his jokes. I'm suspicious because there is no evidence that Jesus ever laughed, and I find that highly unlikely.

Think of all the social events he attended: weddings, dinners with Mary and Martha, dinners with the tax collectors and prostitutes, gathering little children unto himself. Jesus would have to be clinically depressed not to be laughing and joking with this bunch. And how about those Pharisees? Talk about ripe for parody. In my mind there is no question. Jesus was definitely a jokester.

I took the cancer seriously, but didn't want to take myself too seriously. That's why it helps to have a Divine Jester around—although I've had some serious words with Him about that hair.

Mom

Unlike me, my mother has seen cancer done only two ways, both of which resulted in profound wasting and death. She was too scared to be around either of these people, so she missed some of the gifts that can come from being with the terminally ill. She saw them newly diagnosed and then just before they died. So to her, cancer equals death—zero-to-sixty in ten seconds.

I don't think she really understood that cancer is not a death sentence. It's more like a reminder notice—"Just a note to remind you that your time is limited."

I grew up hearing my mother explain death this way, "You die and then the worms eat you."

She had said this breezily in her thirties and forties, but when she started seeing people nearer her own age die, she stopped saying it at all. The Worm Theory is not that attractive to begin with, and is even less so when you apply it to yourself.

When I was a child my mother declared herself an atheist. I have since heard her mention God, so I'm not so sure now. Although both her parents were Spanish, and most of her family was Catholic, she and her brothers and sister were not raised in the Church. That was one reason she didn't believe in God.

The other reason was my illness as an infant. My belly swelled up so that by the time I was nine months old, I looked pregnant. My pediatrician told my mother it was gas. It turned out to be a four-pound tumor attached to my liver. It was benign, but my mother was furious that this God she didn't believe in could let an innocent baby get so sick. So then she *really* didn't believe in God.

My dad, on the other hand, struck a deal with the Big Guy. "Save her life, and I'll take her to church every Sunday."

God said, "Deal." So my dad kept his promise. Every Sunday he took both me and my sister to church. (I think his decision to include my sister was some sort of illness protection plan.)

My mom stayed home and read the paper. My father tried to get her to come, but she wouldn't. Not even on Christmas or Easter. We always celebrated these holidays: church services, big Christmas dinners, Easter dresses, Easter hats, and Easter egg hunts. We just never talked about the true significance of the holidays. My mom was mad at God, didn't believe in God, and she would have nothing to do with Him. So there.

When my mom told me that she was going in to see her doctor to discuss the results of her biopsy, I knew immediately that she had cancer. If your test results are benign, they will tell you over the phone. Doctors don't have you come in unless it's malignant or you're one of those patients who always brings freshly baked cookies or homemade hooch.

I immediately e-mailed an aunt and asked her to accompany my mom. "No matter what she says, go with her. And please take notes," I wrote. My father could have gone, but I was afraid he would be as shocked as Mom and regret that he didn't force her into attending church, perhaps avoiding this disease.

Having my aunt along turned out to be a good idea as my mother completely fell apart and didn't hear a thing. In fact, in our first conversation she kept saying, "I have SIDS! I have SIDS!"

I said, "Mother, you can't have Sudden Infant Death Syndrome."

"That what the doctor said, C-I-D-S."

Ductal Carcinoma In Situ. DCIS. She had the right letters, but in the wrong order.

Knowing how freaked out she was about her diagnosis I dreaded telling her mine. I really tried to downplay it, but it was like trying to downplay "holocaust," or "nuclear attack." As much as having cancer herself scared the hell out of her, she was even more scared for me, and I could hear the pain in her voice.

To know that I was causing my mom's pain—again—was torture for me. I've always felt some irrational guilt over having that tumor when I was a baby. It was a big horrible event for both my parents, and even years later it was hard for them to talk about it.

Then when I was nine, I fell and broke off my two front teeth. This resulted in countless trips to the dentist and orthodontist. At thirteen I had a mole on my nose that my doctor got squirrelly about, and that was another surgery. Growing up it felt as if I was just one big walking problem who cost my parents lots of money. After I worked as a chaplain in pediatrics I realized that I was monstrously healthy compared to a lot of kids.

But talking to my mom on the phone that day I felt such grief over her grief. There is this amazing ping-pong suffering that occurs between a patient and a family member—which brings me to my husband.

Wes

If you ask him now, he'll tell you that he was in total denial for quite a while. When I had my first biopsy, he smiled and said cheerfully, "You've had biopsies before and they've always been negative!"

"I have a feeling," I said.

He didn't like hearing that because my "feelings" are usually right on. Because he is a scientist, and there haven't been any studies on my "feelings," it was easy for him to dismiss this one. But the biggest reason he didn't believe it is because he really, really, really didn't want me to have cancer.

He told me that he felt bad that I had all those biopsies, and now I had to have a mastectomy. I knew he felt bad, and I felt bad that he felt bad. You can see how this ping-pong suffering starts.

The temptation is to start lying about how you feel. We actually had this conversation:

Deb: "Oh, it's no big deal. Just a boob—don't feel bad for me. I'm fine."

Wes: "Oh, I don't feel bad. I'm fine, too."

Then we both burst out laughing because we knew we were such *liars*! We were also laughing because we have an alternate definition of "fine," which was perfectly true.

I once worked with teenagers in recovery, and whenever I said I was "fine," they would say, "FINE: Fucked up, Insecure, Neurotic, and Emotional." That pretty much sums up how you feel when you or a loved one gets cancer.

The only way to stop ping-pong suffering is to simply accept that you *and* your loved ones feel shitty about this whole thing. Period. So feel shitty, move on, and pretty soon you'll all be feeling *fine*.

Wes thought about me dying from this, but he said he knew if he was thinking about me dying, then he wasn't enjoying the present moment in which I was living. So he pretty much worked on staying in the present. He said he knew the statistics and for my kind of tumor, the cure rate was very high. He felt very confident about this.

But at night, he would cry in his sleep. He sounded like a very small child. I didn't want to wake him up, so I would gently rub his back until he stopped crying. I didn't tell him about this for months. When I finally did, he said, "I'm glad I was working it out in my dreams."

For the first month after my diagnosis, we would wake up, and one of us would ask the other, "Did you have that same nightmare that I had? The one where you/I have breast cancer?"

It didn't seem real to either of us for a long time.

Death

Almost everyone who gets a cancer diagnosis starts thinking about death. Even though my surgeon told me that my cancer was curable, I still started thinking about death. This was not new for me since I worked in hospice for many years, and death is pretty much unavoidable there. I've thought about my own death a lot over the years, but after my diagnosis it seemed so much more possible, so much less theoretical.

Death is one of my favorite subjects, but most Americans don't like to think about death or talk about death, let alone actually do it. I've learned the hard way that you can't talk to just anyone about it. Try bringing up death at a dinner party.

"So what do *you* think happens when you die?" It's a total conversation stopper. And Wes loves to talk about *his* work: infectious diseases and parasites. So we just don't get invited out anymore.

A few years ago, some of the medical staff at the Seattle Cancer Care Alliance came to me and said, "We're not comfortable talking to our patients about terminal illness, spirituality, and death." Many of them found themselves wanting to run out of the room, starting to cry, or asking if the patient would like more pudding.

I know it seems crazy that medical staff would be uncomfortable with death. I mean, they see death all the time, right? The truth is, despite the medical school classes about death and dying, physicians still see death as the enemy. Take a look at the mottos of some big cancer centers.

"Working together to cure cancer." (Seattle Cancer Care Alliance)

"Where the power of knowledge saves lives." (City of Hope National Medical Center)

"Fighting cancer is all we do. All day. Every day." (Fox Chase Cancer Center)

"Today's discoveries—tomorrow's cures." (Wistar Institute)

These are all good mottos. Who wants to go to a cancer center that proclaims, "Hoping to make you feel better"? Or "Taking good care of you even if you die"? But notice how insidious this is—everyone wants to fight, cure, and save lives. Death means they've failed.

I knew that until the staff explored their own feelings about death, they couldn't be comfortable talking with their patients. So I created this program called "The Existential Expedition." We didn't want to sound *religious* or anything.

At the first session we talked about our childhood dreams, our family beliefs around pain and suffering in the world, and what called us to the work we're now doing. Each session was two hours, and each group could be no larger than six people. I mean, these are heavy questions and people need time to think, discuss, try on new ideas, and ask questions.

For the second session we talked about spiritual beliefs—what we were raised to believe and what we now believe. People often equate religion with spirituality, and because many staff were not churchgoers, they were surprised to realize that they actually *had* spiritual beliefs.

I think your religion is simply the basket in which you carry your spirituality. So maybe you carry your spirituality in a Jewish basket, a Buddhist basket, an Islamic basket, a Christian basket, or a basket without a name. Whatever. The important thing is that you don't get more hooked on the basket than the contents.

The contents involve life's meaning, how it can be cherished and nourished. It's about how you cope with life, how you view it, how you experience it, where you find meaning. There is a lot of common ground between religions when you look at them under the broader umbrella of "spirituality."

But anyway, about "The Existential Expedition": we saved the best for last. At the final session we talked about what we thought about death. Keep in mind that the group had already spent four hours together sharing their beliefs. Every discussion included lots of laughter, a fair amount of tears, and copious amounts of Diet Coke and coffee.

The first question was, what do you think happens when you die? Personally, I've thought about this a lot. I like to try on different ideas about death. The Heaven and Hell thing just doesn't work for me. Perhaps it's the heavenly fashions that bug me. If you're going to get some perfect new body, why cover it up with all that fabric? And why the sandals? Heaven for me would mean comfortable heels.

So sometimes I think, well, what if it's like we're ocean waves? You know, you take a snapshot of a wave, and then you go back the next day and that particular wave is gone, but the ocean's still there. So where's the wave? It still exists, right? It's just not in the same form.

Or what if it's like the Buddhists say that you come here to learn something, and if you don't get it this time, you have to reincarnate, and try it again? But if you've managed to learn it then you can stay in nirvana or you can *choose* to come back as a bodhisattva, and help the rest of us. I love that idea. I mean, haven't you met people, especially children, and said to yourself, "Hmm, you've been here before, haven't you?"

Or what if after we die we'll be backstage saying to one another, "Oh, my God, you were so good as the overbearing mother! And you, you were the cranky checkout guy—fantastic!" What if we're all playing parts?

I really don't know. Someone told me death is whatever you believe it to be. And I thought, "Well, which day?" I just know we could all do each other a big favor by being more open and curious, instead of avoiding talking about it.

So here was the final question of "The Existential Expedition": if you had to die right now, how would you want to die? I gave them all sorts of choices: drowning, murder, heart failure, house fire, Alzheimer's disease, shark attack, car accident, snake bite, or poison mushrooms. I knew I had to offer lots of choices because of my experience in hospice. I would often hear patients saying, "Oh, w-a-a-a-h, I'm dying of cancer."

And I'd say, "Yes, that's right. How did you want to die?" That would always stop them in their tracks, because they never thought about it. So here was the most surprising thing: more than seventy oncology staff went through this program, and 80 percent of them chose cancer as a way they would like to die.

One nurse said, "Before this group, I would have said that cancer is the worst. But after really thinking and talking about it, which I never did before now, I see that cancer can give you time to say goodbye, thank you, and I love you. It gives your family some time to get used to the fact that you are going to die."

"That is so true!" another said. "Sudden death is horrible for your family. My brother died suddenly, and it was so unbelievable. I kept waiting for him to call me or send me a damn postcard. It took me a year to really get that he was dead. Then I started grieving. So I would pick cancer."

Still another said, "I can't believe I'm going to say this, but I choose cancer, too. My big fear was pain, but I know from experience we can control most cancer pain with medication."

No one chose death by murder or car accident: too violent. A house fire: too painful. Drowning: too scary. Poison mushrooms: too . . . embarrassing.

So if 80 percent chose cancer as how they would like to die, what did the other 20 percent choose? The old standby: they wanted to die in their sleep—with the house clean, the laundry done, and the refrigerator full.

Oh, yeah—how did *I* choose to die?

Cancer.

Two

RATS!

Dear Family and Friends,

Well, Wes and I would rather have a rat invasion than a cancer invasion (although some have told us rats are harder to get rid of), but we don't have a choice in the matter.

My pathology report came back, and I was tempted to return it immediately and write NOT ACCEPTABLE on it. It turns out that one of my nodes was positive. I must say, Wes and I were absolutely stunned. I actually felt that this mastectomy was quite doable and I'd be back at work in a few weeks. Well, now it's a whole new ball game.

Also, although we are both mightily in favor of coach to first class airline upgrades, we are *not* happy that my tumor was upgraded from grade I to grade II. That little overachiever!

We found this out on Tuesday night, and I would have let you know sooner, but I've been busy trying to breathe. Plus, there is, as of yet, no treatment plan. The Breast Cancer Specialty Clinic (and delicatessen) meets Tuesday to discuss my case. We don't see an oncologist for another week after that. So we are in that sucky No Clue Zone.

I am not in favor of chemo for two major reasons: (1) I just got these highlights done, and (2) I have a really unattractive flat spot/indentation on the back of my head. Seriously, it's big enough for a birdbath. So chemo doesn't excite me—although I've heard that all that vomiting really strengthens the core muscles.

I am not in favor of radiation because isn't that how Godzilla got started? Wasn't it some sort of radiation accident? I think I carry that GDZL-2 gene.

And as for further node dissection—ever notice how the word "die" is embedded in that phrase? I can hardly lift my arm now, and they took out only three nodes! So I say, "No way nodes!"

I guess that leaves voodoo. I'll have to research that.

My mom's lumpectomy is Monday morning, and I haven't told her any of this. She is already sick with worry, and I don't think she needs to go into surgery with this crappy news. In fact, I was thinking of telling her my mastectomy was really a C-section, and she has twin grandchildren! She would be so happy! She would probably have a spontaneous miracle healing.

The most fun I've had this week was calling my patients. They were happy to update me with their news and to give me advice. Honestly—it was so great, a win-win situation. I'm telling everyone at work to be open about me having breast cancer. If they simply say, "She's out for a month," the patients will be thinking I'm in jail for shoplifting or God-knows-what. And, I'm happy to be the poster child for yearly mammograms.

Okay, dear friends, that's all for now. Thanks again for all your love and support. Also, don't hesitate to call. We have an answering machine, so if I can't talk to you, I won't answer, and you can leave a message. Or you can e-mail me: Debra@debrajarvis.com.

But don't feel that you have to keep in touch.

Just know that you'll be out of the will if you don't.

Love and Hugs,
Debra

P.S. I've thought of the title of my next book: *This Sucks! What to Say, How To Be, and What To Do When Your Friend Has Cancer.* This is based on my recent personal experience of well-meaning friends saying unbelievably stupid and hurtful things. The only thing that has kept me from homicide is: they weren't close enough to shoot, and (the real reason) I know that their intentions were good.

Still Speaking

It was a few days after my diagnosis, and I had just arrived at work, walking down the hall, slightly preoccupied with the fact that I, myself, had cancer, when I heard this noise that immediately made me think of a documentary I saw about hyenas. Hyenas aren't sitting around laughing and telling jokes. They make that maniacal sound when they are being submissive. But I could tell that whoever was in room 31, a room with a door, was not being submissive. She was being abusive.

"You don't understand! I have *cancer*! You couldn't possibly understand!" If we get a heads-up from a case manager that a patient may be "high maintenance," we put them in a room with a door, if available, until things calm down.

She was shrieking and crying, and a man was sitting in an upholstered chair next to her bed. As I walked by and looked through the window, I could see that he kept trying to hold her hand, and she would shake him off. She was a first dose patient, so of course, I'd stop by and say hi. Her name was Charlotte.

Besides the verbal conversation with a patient, there is another level of communication that goes on, and for lack of a better word, I'll call it the energetic level. I think part of my job is to balance the energy during the encounter. This means that if someone is in high drama, maybe near hysterics, I'll go into the room so laid-back, you'd think I'd been lying on the beach sipping margaritas all day.

Speaking of beverages, I'll bring in a cup of tea, because there is something really grounding about that. Clearly a visit to room 31 called for strong Earl Grey with milk. Some patients call for green chai, others for cocoa spice. Still others Jack Daniels, but that's not allowed.

The tea is not only for me. I've found that watching me drink tea helps patients calm down a little. I mean it can't be that bad if the chaplain is sipping tea.

I drink my tea in a red commuter cup, which let's face it, is an adult sippy cup. On one side of my cup it says, "United Church of Christ." On the other side it has a big black comma with the words, "God is still speaking." The comma refers to the Gracie Allen quote, "Never place a period where God has placed a comma." Maybe Gracie was referring to our church forefather John Robinson.

When the Pilgrims were leaving Europe with Mayflower Moving to invent Thanksgiving in Massachusetts, John Robinson sent them off with this sound bite: "God has yet more light and truth to break forth out of his holy Word."

This means to me that there is no once-and-for-all interpretation of scripture. I know as absolute truth Mr. Martha Miyagi never stops talking. It's just a matter of whether or not I'm able to hear. Maybe next year they'll come up with a cup that says, "Keep listening."

Anyway, I knocked on the door of room 31, set down my tea, and washed my hands. "Hi, Charlotte? I'm Debra, the general oncology chaplain—just dropped by to say hi."

"You're the chaplain?" she asked before breaking into the hyena sobbing again. She was in her sixties, and her hair was dyed a little too dark so that it gave her a harsh look. I could see her foundation coming off on her tissue.

The man in the chair stood up, and we shook hands. "Hi, I'm her husband, Ed."

I sat down on a rolling stool and scooted up to her bed. I let her howl for a little bit and then, this is how laid-back I got: I yawned. I mean, it wasn't a fake yawn, I *really* yawned, and my eyes started to tear up, like when you first get up in the morning. I dispensed with the usual concierge questions. Wiping my eyes and sniffing, I asked, "So what's happening?" If I got any more laid-back I would have been rolling a joint.

"I. Have. Cancer."

For a moment I thought about yawning again and saying, "Yeah, me too." But instead I reached over and squeezed her arm and said, "Then you are in the right place."

She wasn't crying anymore. "Colon. Cancer," she said.

"So what are we giving you today?" I asked this question because it gives me a clue to how involved a patient is in his or her medical care. If she put her hands over her face and said, "Oh, God, I don't know," then I would know that she was probably too fearful to find out.

But she said, "I'm getting 5-FU and oxaliplatin for six months and then surgery."

Okay, so she was informed. I sipped my tea. "So tell me how all this came about."

Her story was that her cancer was found early on a routine colonoscopy. This was good news.

"If you think getting a tube stuck up your ass is easy, let me tell you . . ."

"You were sedated," Ed said. "You're weren't even awake."

She ignored him. "Well, the real fun is the bowel prep. They make you drink this *stuff*, it's ghastly, and then you have diarrhea for *hours*."

I could tell that she was going down a well-trod verbal path. She had probably told this story a hundred times. Her husband excused himself. While she went on with her story, always just this side of hysterical, I sipped my tea and waited.

I was listening to her, and there was an energetic undercurrent of thoughts humming through me: no drama necessary. It's only cancer. It's only death. What's death? Just the closing of the circle. No big deal.

The Dalai Lama is often seen laughing and smiling. Lighten up, he seems to be saying. This too shall pass. The United Church of Christ has ads that read, "If you think getting up on Sunday mornings is hard, try rising from the dead." Lighten up.

What does the dramatic emotion get you? Attention from others, at a time when what you really need is attention from yourself. Pay attention to yourself, and you won't need it so much from everyone else. This was all going on at that energetic level I was talking about.

When she came back around to retelling the bowel prep story I interrupted.

"Charlotte, your prognosis is good. So what do you make of all this?"

"What do I *make* of it? Well, I guess I'm not surprised."

"Why are you not surprised?"

This is when she went from hyena to bunny. This is what I was waiting for.

"Well, my dad died of colon cancer when I was in high school. Then Mom was diagnosed with breast cancer a few years after that. She died just before I graduated from college."

"How sad that she didn't get to see you graduate."

She just nodded because she was crying very quietly into her tissue. "I knew I would get cancer. How could I not?" I handed her another tissue.

Her prognosis was good, but like my mom, all she knew was that cancer equals death. She probably didn't even hear her oncologist tell her that her cancer was curable.

"You have no idea what it's like to have parents with cancer, and then get cancer yourself."

"Yes."

I meant, "Yes, I do," but she didn't know that, and it didn't really matter. I stayed a little longer, and she told me about growing up in the Episcopal Church, and how she found it cold.

"Ah, yes, the 'frozen chosen.'"

That made her laugh, and before I left she squeezed my hand and said, "Thank you for coming."

"You're welcome. Can I bring you anything—a cup of tea?"

"That would be perfect."

Food for the Journey

I kept telling myself that this whole cancer thing was no big deal. So it seemed to me that the logical thing to do was to prepare for my surgery by cooking and cleaning. I made a big pot of chicken-vegetable soup. Little did I know at the time I was chopping vegetables that these would be the last things I chopped for months.

I've always believed that cooking food is both mystical and magical. When I cook for parties and dinners, I think of who is going to be at our table. I visualize each person and say a little prayer for them as I'm slicing or sautéing. So I prayed for myself and Wes.

It's tempting to say, "Especially for Wes," which would make me sound all unselfish and saintly, but it isn't true. I think it's a big mistake not to pray for yourself. You know, it's the whole put-your-oxygen-on-first-and-then-you-can-assist-others deal.

Since I've given you my take on Jesus, I should give you my take on prayer. I don't think God is Santa Claus. You know, you hand God a list and hope the list is checked twice and you'll get what you asked for based on whether you've been naughty or nice.

If you ask me to pray for you, I don't ask the Divine to do this or that. Instead, I visualize you surrounded by Light. I visualize you so at peace and feeling the spiritual presence of Mr. Martha Miyagi that whatever happens you will remain at peace.

One of the best e-mails I received after my diagnosis was from a Quaker friend who wrote, "I am fervently holding you in the Light." Nothing about curing, nothing about making events go a certain way. And whenever I felt exhausted or sick, I remembered that I was being held, "in the Light." Fervently. I felt comforted, loved, protected.

So as I chopped carrots and broccoli, onions and garlic, I visualized myself and Wes surrounded by the Light. I saw us eating this good soup and feeling at peace. As I cut up the chicken I whispered, "I hope you had a good chicken life—laid a few eggs, hatched some chicks, maybe had some grandchicks. Sorry about the decapitation. I hope you enjoy being in my soup. Thank you, thank you, thank you."

To be honest, I don't always commune with my food in quite this way, but the days leading up to my surgery had a Last Supper quality to them that made everything seem Significant and Important. This was because we knew nothing would ever be the same.

Things would be different after my mastectomy, but it didn't mean things would be bad. It would be up to me to figure out how to accept things as different and not worse.

Calling All Patients

Even though I told my colleagues that it was perfectly okay, and they had my express permission to share my diagnosis with my patients, I knew it would be hard for them. We've all been HIPAA-cized to death and are terrified of accidentally sharing medical information. HIPAA, or the Health Insurance Portability and Accountability Act, or the "Keep Your Big Mouth Shut Act," is basically a good thing. It keeps medical information super private and confidential, and we all learned not to talk about patients in front of other patients, in the elevator, in the hallways, or in the restroom. (You never know who is the next stall.) If we receive a written message with a patient's name on it, when we're done with it we have to either throw it in a special recycling box or eat it.

So I knew that asking the nurses to tell my patients I was home recovering from a mastectomy was like asking them to drink poison. I realized I needed to call my patients myself. I had been seeing some of these people for months, so for me to just suddenly drop off the face of the earth with no explanation seemed downright rude.

I made a list and a latte and started dialing. Don't think I wasn't a little nervous about this. For one thing, I wasn't making the call from the clinic. I was sitting in my kitchen in my sweatshirt and jeans, and I didn't feel very professional. My plan was to simply say I'd be back at work in six weeks, and another chaplain would be visiting.

In chaplaincy training we are taught to keep the focus of the conversation on the patient. We learn to listen reflectively, which is basically feeding back to someone what we hear him or her saying. That is why chaplains can be such good party guests—we are trained to be fabulous listeners, which makes other people think we are great conversationalists.

Of course, sometimes the reverse is true. A chaplain will go to a party and think, "I'm not at work. Now I can talk about me, me, *me!*" and then all we do is drone on about ourselves. Forgive us. Simply tell us about some minor tragedy in your life and we'll snap out of it. We can't help it. At one party I stopped in the middle of telling a story because I saw a woman's eyes filling with tears.

"What's going on?" I asked softly. She just shook her head and waved me off. I put my hand on her arm. "No, really. You can tell me."

She pointed to a huge tabby who was sitting on the couch licking itself. "I'm allergic to that goddamn cat."

So my first instinct when making these phone calls was to tell them my news and then get the conversation back to how they were doing. But this was not to be. I felt as if I called the mastectomy hotline.

"Oh, my God! Did they give you stool softeners? Take extra with a big glass of water and eat an apple a day. Fruit will save your ass and I mean that literally."

"Start your arm stretching as soon as you can. I'll send you my exercise sheet. And soups—soups are quite good for you, keep you hydrated. Be conscientious about taking senna with every pain pill."

"You're gonna be sleeping on your back, okay? So honey, here's what you need to do: get one of those knee wedges so you don't get back pain. Are they giving you stool softeners?"

It's known that people tend to regress when they have serious illnesses, and to be sure, when you are going through surgery and chemo you may as well be a newborn, because it's all about eating and pooping. Especially pooping because pain medication can constipate the hell out of you. So I received lots of advice about that.

At first I was uncomfortable with this, but I saw that allowing people to help me was empowering for them. When you are a patient and receiving so much care from everyone, it's easy to feel as if you have no value. This is especially true if you are used to being effective, efficient, and competent. Not only were our phone conversations a chance for them to give me excellent advice, it also deepened our relationship. I realized once again that we connect through our vulnerabilities, not our strengths. That is why when you encounter severe turbulence on a plane flight, you may feel closer to your seatmate than to your own grandmother.

The Heart of the Matter

Even though I had been seeing him for months, Haruki Ito was a bit of a mystery to me. He never failed to be polite, as was his wife, Michiko. He was diagnosed with lymphoma, and for a long time just cruised along with it. But suddenly everything went out of control with his white blood cells, and that's how I met him, when he came in for chemotherapy.

He was a well-known painter who had taught for many years in a well-known art school. Both he and his wife were born in Japan, and even though they had lived for many years in the United States, they had the ingrained habit of bowing ever so slightly whenever I greeted them. It was as if there was an accent to their body language.

As polite as they always were, they were also very private about their feelings and their stories. I knew they had no children, and I could see they were devoted to one another. It would be easy to describe them as "cold" and "distant" except I felt nothing but warmth from them.

They both were always neat and well groomed. Michiko often wore jeans with high heel boots. Her hair was perfectly cut into a shiny black bob. Haruki wore carefully ironed white shirts and pressed jeans.

I gave them lots of space to tell their stories, but I ended up learning more about them on Google than I did by talking with them. The notes in his chart were vague when it came to "social history." It seemed Haruki's doctor didn't have any better luck than I did. If any couple acted as though cancer was no big deal, it was the Itos.

Any attempts to discuss his worsening disease or their spiritual beliefs were skillfully and politely parried. So we talked about art and music and sushi. I scored big with them when I told them I had my first sashimi at age thirteen when my sixth grade teacher took us to the Ginza Café in downtown San Jose, California. I kept visiting because they always said before I left, "Thank you for coming to speak with us. Please come back." So I did.

But it was clear the usual chemo and then the experimental chemo wasn't working. Haruki grew thin and weak until at last he was hospitalized. I went to see him in the hospital a few days before my surgery. When I arrived, I was shocked to find Haruki was in a coma and on a ventilator. Michiko sat quietly in a chair right next to his bed. She was wearing her signature jeans, boots, and a pink turtleneck. I sat down next to her and put my arm around her. I had only shaken her hand before, but this felt like the right thing to do.

"He is going to get better," she said.

I didn't tell her that his nurse grabbed me in the hall to tell me that his blood pressure was dropping, and he was having kidney failure and wouldn't make it another twenty-four hours.

There was nothing to say to her. I couldn't suggest prayer, or ask her if she would like me to read scripture to her. So I simply sat with my arm around her.

The attending physician came in, and I could tell he was waiting for me to leave before he spoke to her when Michiko said, "You can talk in front of Debra. She is a friend." I was touched and felt my throat tighten.

He tried, as did the nurse and resident after him, to make her understand that Haruki was dying. "He has multiple organ failure. That means his vital organs are shutting down, and there is nothing we can do to stop it."

"Give him a more powerful drug."

"There isn't a more powerful drug. We can't give him any more Lasix—it's not working. He is not responding to anything."

"Please do everything."

The attending was quiet for a while and then reached out and took her hand. "We'll do what we can, Mrs. Ito."

I knew their thirty-fifth wedding anniversary was coming up. In fact, it was on the day of my surgery. So I asked her, "Michiko, are you trying to keep Haruki alive until your anniversary?"

"No, I am just waiting for him to wake up."

I let a lot of silence settle around us before I asked, "Michiko, what do you believe happens when you die?"

"I don't know. Nothing."

She did not have faith in anything beyond herself, anything that could comfort her now or later. No sense of a bigger picture. And where were their friends?

"Are your friends coming?"

She sighed and wiped her eyes. "We have told no one. Haruki did not want anyone to know." Her mascara was smeared, her perfect bob a mess. She took both my hands in hers. "You must understand that in our culture we do not tell people outside of the family our problems. It was difficult for us to tell you things. And now, I want a miracle. But from where, Debra? I don't believe in miracles." Then she got up and went over to the bed. She bent over Haruki, crying and tenderly speaking to him in Japanese while the ventilator swished and moaned.

"When he dies it will be as if your arm is cut off," I said.

"No. It is my heart. My heart will be cut out."

When I got home that night I said to Wes, "If anything happens on the table and I end up on a ventilator and the prognosis is bad, give me three days. That's it. If I can't figure out how to come back in three days, I'm not supposed to come back."

Haruki died the next day, and I never told Michiko about my surgery.

Looking the Part

During my pre-op appointment, I was told that the thing to do was to get a mastectomy camisole. So the day before my surgery, I swung into Nordstrom. My eyes instantly went to the dresses, the shoes, and the cosmetics. But that was not what I was there for. My mission: find the camisole. I made my way to the lingerie department. Would they be hanging on a rack?

The first things I saw were all the lacey teddies and the sexy bras with matching panties. I love that stuff. That is when I felt my throat close up and a burning sensation in my eyes. I fingered a red satin push-up bra while I blinked back my tears. I wanted to go back in time, before the biopsy, before the mammogram. I wanted to be able to place my little breasts in that red push-up bra, and go to a party. That's it—I wanted a party, not a mastectomy. I finally pulled myself together and approached the salesgirl who I judged to be around thirteen.

Please understand that I never pay retail. So when she told me the camisole was fifty dollars I nearly choked.

"I don't suppose they ever go on sale, do they?"

Her eyes got really wide, and she handed me the box and said, "This is the smallest size we have."

It was white and made of the softest cotton knit I've ever touched. It had soft feminine lace around the neckline and a sort of peplum at the bottom. Everything about it screamed, "No sex! Can't you see I've just had surgery?"

But there were two really cool things about it: (1) the neck was wide enough so that you could step into it, and (2) there were two pockets in the front on each side. These were for your drains. Hideous, but true, I'd have a drain coming out of my surgery site. Usually you'd pin the drain onto your pants, and then when you needed to pee, you'd forget about the bulb and pull down your pants and yank on your drain. Or, you could pin it to your shirt, but then you'd have that clammy rubber bulb touching your skin. (In the hospital they pinned it inside my gown, and it felt like some creepy little hand trying to cop a feel.)

The camisole even came with a fake boob. It looked enormous to me, but the salesgirl explained that you removed the stuffing until it matched your other breast. I knew I was getting a saline implant at the time of my mastectomy, so I didn't bother with getting the prosthesis down to size. I was afraid I'd be sitting there all day tearing out stuffing.

The step-in camisole reminded me that I wouldn't want to be reaching over my head and putting on and taking off clothes. I was wandering through the mall, wondering what to wear with my new camisole when I found myself in the sportswear section of JCPenney. And there, *on sale*, were these really light, soft warm-up suits—*drawstring* pants and *zip-up* jacket. That meant no yanking down waistbands or reaching over my head! And these suits were soft enough to sleep in but were made for the daytime.

Yes, Grasshopper, seek and ye shall find on sale.

I immediately bought two, one aqua blue and one black for those dress-up occasions like dinner in the kitchen versus dinner in bed.

The last store I visited on my pre-op shopping trip was the Body Shop. I'm not sure why I was drawn there because the irony of the store name was not lost on me, but the minute I walked in, I knew why.

Sitting there looking up at me with huge golden-brown eyes was a beautiful ginger-colored dog with sticky-uppy ears. He was on a leash, and his mistress was yakking with the salesgirl and didn't even notice me squat down and pet him. He snuggled right up to me and kissed my face all over. And then it was as if this faucet that I had kept tightly closed burst open. I started crying with silent hiccupping sobs. He kept licking my face, licking all the tears that were rolling down my cheeks. When he was satisfied that the flow was slowing down, he turned over on his back, and I scratched his belly. This got the attention of his owner who looked down and exclaimed, "Oh, gosh! He never does that for anyone. He must think you're special."

I just kept scratching his belly and said, "Oh, no, I think he just knew I needed some dog energy today."

I didn't want her to see me crying. I wanted to say, "I want to wear those cute lacey push-up bras, but I had to buy a grandma garment because tomorrow they're taking off my breast and my dog died three years ago, and where is she now that I really need her? And I guess I'm a little more scared than I thought since I'm squatting here in the Body Shop of all places, and your dog is making me feel safe and loved and telling me that everything is going to be okay, and it's these little acts of kindness, these subtle, small, surprising signs of love, that make me cry." But I thought saying all that might freak her out.

Instead, I bent down and kissed him on his forehead, on that smooth part just between and above his brows. Then I quietly got up and walked out. The woman holding the leash never noticed.

I cried my way out of the mall and out to my car, now and then raising my hand to my face so I could smell the dog's scent still on my hands. Did I think I would get through this without ever crying? Sure I was familiar with breast cancer, but I wasn't familiar with *my* breast cancer.

It was no big deal and it *was* a big deal. It was both/and, not either/or. It was messy and mushy and mixed up. Lighten up and take it seriously.

I was exhausted by the time I got home, but I laid out my clothes and inspected them. I always do this with new clothes: lay them out and imagine with what and where I will wear them. No big puzzle—I'd wear them to and from the hospital and at home recuperating. The only problem I could see with these ensembles is that the pants were at least four inches too long.

Now, let me stop here and say that as soon as my friends and neighbors heard I had cancer, almost everyone of them said, "Let me know if there is anything I can do." People truly want to do something because they love you and feel so helpless.

I've heard countless patients tell me how they turned down offers of dinner, babysitting, rides, lawn mowing, house cleaning, and free theatre tickets. They would say this proudly as if turning down their friends and family was some godly act of profound virtue.

If I know they are Christians, I'll bring up the story of Peter going ape-shit because Jesus wants to wash the disciples' feet. I know there are all kinds of symbolic meanings to that passage, but on one level, what I hear Jesus saying to Peter is, "Get over your pride and self-sufficiency."

When patients say, "Oh, no, I don't want to bother anyone."

I ask, "Can you see how letting your friends help you is also a gift to *them*?"

So I called up my next-door neighbor who is wicked good on the serger. She came over right away. "Mary," I said, "could you please hem these two pair of pants for me?"

"Sure," she said. "I'll get them to you by the weekend."

"No, I need them for my mastectomy tomorrow."

She didn't miss a beat. "No problem."

I was pretty proud of myself because I have my own serger and technically could have done it myself. But psychically, I didn't have room for one more thing.

Running Away and Pushing Up

Was I nervous before my surgery? Not really—I was too busy. I wasn't due at the hospital until four o'clock that afternoon. I was well aware that I wouldn't be jogging anytime soon after surgery, so Wes and I decided to go on a five-mile run. It felt quite surreal. We both knew that this was the last time we would ever run like this together. Not the last time we would run together, just the last time *like this*—whole and without regard for my right breast—because it would be gone.

It was a gorgeous day, Cinco de Mayo, May 5, my grandmother's birthday. She would have been ninety-three had she not died the year before. She had never had a mammogram in her life. Yeah, the mother and grandmother of two women with breast cancer. Go figure.

After the run, we stretched, and I did fifteen full push-ups. I'd never done that many before, and so far, have not again. Then I did a yoga headstand. And a handstand. I did cartwheels on the lawn in the backyard. I hung from a tree branch. I held a backbend for two full minutes.

"Are you auditioning for Cirque du Soleil?" Wes asked.

"No," I grunted while clasping my hands behind my back and attempting to lift them over my head. "I'm doing all the things I know I won't be doing for a while."

He just nodded, came over, and kissed me on my sweaty neck.

A Clean Breast of Things

I've talked to women who have done elaborate rituals before their mastectomies: wrote songs and poems about their breasts, took photos of them, lit candles. For many women their breasts are a huge part of their identity. Mine were neither huge nor an important part of my identity.

Here is what I did just before surgery: I looked down at the right one, which by this time was quite bruised and upset looking. I got in the shower, took the Hibiclens, and washed my breast, armpit, and chest area as instructed.

I dried myself with a clean towel as instructed. I then turned to Wes and said, "Last look! Show closes at four o'clock!"

He said something like, "Honey, that breast has got some badness in it and it's better that you take it off." It wasn't that he was afraid to say, "cancer," it was just that we were sick of hearing the word.

"Yes," I said, "I believe that's biblical: If thy breast offends thee cut it off."

So we were both in pretty good moods on the way to the hospital. My mood changed once I got into that skanky hospital gown, and they wouldn't let me wear any underpants. Then a nurse walked me down this long hall past a bunch of construction workers. Construction workers!

Did I mention I wasn't wearing any underpants? Construction workers have panty *radar*. So I knew they knew I was panty-less; that I was in the midst of a panty famine; that I was overdrawn at the panty bank; that I was *sans culotte*; that I was pantieopenic; that I was thong-less in Seattle. It was at this point that I realized exactly how nervous I was.

I wanted drugs. Specifically I wanted what in the olden days were called "tranquilizers," but now they're all uptown about it and call them "anti-anxiety medications." But I hadn't yet signed the consent form, so I couldn't have any. I did not get my Ativan (aka Vitamin A) until just before they wheeled me into the operating room, and by that time I was like a feral cat on speed. So my advice? Sign the consent forms ASAP and then as soon as they get an IV in your hand, ask for the Vitamin A or Valium or whatever.

They put me on a gurney the size of a cruise ship, and Wes came with me as far as the doors to the pre-op area. We kissed one another good-bye as if I were simply running out to the store. What else could we do? Would a longer kiss make a difference?

In pre-op they put inflatable stockings on me, which made me feel like the Michelin man, and then they wrapped me up burrito-style in a forced-air warming blanket, as it's like a meat locker in the OR. Oh, yeah, then they put that hideous shower cap thing on me. The last thing I remember is my surgeon looking down on me and asking, "Okay, are you ready to do this?"

"Yup."

So the plan was to remove the breast, nip out a few lymph nodes, and that would be that. I woke up to my surgeon saying, "Your lymph nodes look good!" I smiled and envisioned my nodes as elongated, luminescent pearls connected by a string of diamonds swirling and swaying in a sea of clear and pulsing light. Then they gave me more morphine, and I went back to sleep.

When I awoke again a nurse was standing over me. "If you don't pee I'm going to have to catheterize you," she said.

"But I'm dehydrated," I said. "I ran five miles before my surgery!" I managed to produce enough urine to avoid the catheter. "May I have some water, please?"

She brought the water, I drank it, and I promptly threw up. After that, it was nothing but Wes feeding me ice chips. The next time I peed, I was pleased to see they had cleaned my toilet already. I could tell because it was filled with bright blue toilet cleaner. I liked that they had not only done this quickly, but quietly. I had not even heard anybody come in.

It was only after I used the toilet the *next* time that I realized the bright blue was the color of my urine. I was excreting the dye they had injected into my breast that eventually found its way to my lymph nodes.

I spent only twenty-four hours in the hospital and here's why: Trying to sleep in the hospital is like trying to sleep during an NPR pledge break; like trying to sleep in the middle of Costco on a Saturday; like trying to sleep in a hen house after the fox walks in. In other words: impossible.

Wes drove me home the next afternoon. It was the "Princess and the Pea on Wheels." I felt every bump, rock, and piece of gravel on the road. Every stop I thought I was going to fly through the windshield. Every turn I felt as if I were being thrown against the door or the steering wheel.

"Could you take it a little slower?" I growled. "I think this car needs new shocks." Then I just kept muttering, "New shocks," all the way home. How could I have known I was prophesizing?

Wes drove up to the front door, helped me out of the car, into the bed, and gently kissed me. I fell asleep thinking, "The worst is over now."

We took the big bandages off in forty-eight hours, and then there was nothing but the steri-strips and little pieces of suture sticking out on either end of the incision.

I had a total mastectomy. This is not like slicing off a chunk of baloney. It's more like removing a wallet from a purse. The surgeon makes an incision, an ellipsis in your skin, and then removes your nipple and the breast underneath. Some people thought I was either going to have a round open wound or a circular scar as if I'd been stabbed by a biscuit cutter. I had a four-inch horizontal scar.

Because I had an implant put in at the time of my mastectomy, I had a little mound there, almost the size of my other breast. In fact, in the medical literature, it's called a "breast mound." We found this so amusing that we began using "mound" after everything, as in, "I need to wash my hand mounds," or "Just a minute while I blow my nose mound." But because I had a little something there, I didn't experience the shock that many women do.

Two days later, I was out walking in our nearby park. Sure, I was a little glassy-eyed and hanging onto Wes, but I was out walking. I could see that after my incisions healed, I was going to return to my life. I decided I would be religious about performing my post-op stretching so I could go back to yoga class as soon as possible.

A few days later, we had just finished dinner, and Wes was cleaning up. My laptop was on the kitchen table, so out of curiosity, I decided to go online and read my operative report. It was pretty boring: a lot technical stuff about my "clavipectoral fascia" and "nipple areolar complex." It said nothing about how I looked in that dorky shower cap. Maybe the pathology report was more interesting.

It seemed pretty boring, too. I yelled to Wes over the dishwasher, "They have the audacity to describe my pearl-like lymph nodes as, 'tan-brown!'" We laughed and I scrolled down to the final diagnosis.

"Micrometastatic carcinoma in one of three sentinel lymph nodes."

"What?!" I screamed. Wes dropped the pot he was washing and came to the table and read over my shoulder. He put his arms around me, and I could hear him swallowing.

"It's micrometastases (micromets)," he whispered. "Maybe it's nothing."

My surgeon said my lymph nodes looked good. I fell for it. But how could he possibly tell? They were micromets—he didn't have microscopes at the end of his eyes! But even micromets scared the hell out of me, because I knew that once cancer cells were in my lymph nodes, they could go anywhere. I started sobbing, "I don't want to be in the chemo chair!"

We both sat there staring at the screen, and I cried and cried and cried. Then I stopped because I realized we didn't really know what this meant or what we should do. Welcome to the No Clue Zone.

Wes was so stunned that the next day he called the lab and asked to review the slides with a pathologist. "I just have to see for myself," he said.

When he got home that night I asked, "What did you see?"

"Cancer cells."

No Clue Zone

A few months after I started working at the SCCA I had a new chemo patient say to me, "This is the happiest day of my life."

"What?" I asked incredulously.

She paused for a moment and then said, "Okay, well it's the *second* happiest day of my life. The first was when I finally got diagnosed."

She went on to explain that for months she knew something was wrong, but nobody could figure it out. When at last she was correctly diagnosed with colon cancer, she was thrilled.

"It wasn't that I was happy to have cancer, you understand. It's just that I hated feeling sick and not knowing why. And then once they diagnosed me, they didn't yet know if I should have surgery first or chemo. I needed tests. I had to wait for results. Then my doctors had to decide. I thought I would go crazy."

I understand this now. After the pathology report came back with a positive node, we had to change direction, but which direction? It's like driving on the freeway and realizing you've taken the wrong exit. You have to get back on the freeway and take a different exit, but you don't yet know which one to take. So you're sort of idling on the entrance ramp, imagining all the possible turns.

It's very hard to remain in the present moment when you're in this zone. I wanted direction, I wanted a plan, and let's face it, I wanted *control*. I wanted to know what we were going to do. But the No Clue Zone is not about doing. It's about being.

As often happens, I remembered a conversation I had a few weeks earlier, but this time it was as if I was talking to myself.

A woman came in to talk with me because she couldn't get over her guilt about not seeing her doctor immediately in spite of feeling a lump in her breast. She felt bad about the burden it put upon her family for her to go through chemo and radiation and surgery. They removed all the cancer, and she was considered disease-free. But she was also living in constant fear of a recurrence. She sat across the table from me with her legs crossed, nervously shaking her foot.

"So then you're missing out on whatever is happening in the present," I said.

"What do you mean?" she asked.

"Well, when you are fearful, you're living in the future, right? You aren't living in the past, because you can't fear the past. That's over."

She stopped her nervous foot shaking and nodded, so I continued. "Then when you're feeling guilty, you are living in the past. You can't feel guilty about the future, because you haven't done anything yet."

I could see that she immediately understood what I was talking about. She leaned forward and put her hands on the table. "Okay, I get that. But just how am I supposed to keep myself in the present?"

I knew the answer to this one. I felt like the student who studied for the test and was now getting all the right questions. "You want to stay in your body to keep in the present moment. One way to do that is to check in with your breath. Just notice— in-breath or out-breath? Mouth or nose? Don't try to change anything, just notice. Noticing your breath keeps you in your body and in the present."

Well, she really liked that. And here I was weeks later, taking my own advice—again. I really didn't feel any fear until the All-Star Parade of Possible Future Scenarios came marching by. When I was truly in the present I felt content. This whole "Be here now," thing is old as dirt and tons of people have written about it: Ram Dass, Gary Zukav, Eckhardt Tolle.

I think Jesus was saying the same thing. The disciples are jumping up and down asking, "When is the kingdom of God coming?" They're fantasizing about something they think is way off in the future.

And Jesus says, "The kingdom of God is now."

Of course, this totally bums them out because they are looking forward to the glory of an everlasting all night party. I'm sure when Jesus told them, "In my Father's house are many rooms," they were thinking, "Dude—party!"

Speaking of Jesus, don't think I didn't have a word or two with Mr. Martha Miyagi about this positive node.

"Just what is the point of this? How are you going to use this little development?"

Triple M was curiously silent on this.

So I didn't freak out, but I couldn't help but wonder: Am I going to get chemo? Have more nodes removed? Radiation? And what am I going to tell my mother?

Role Reversal

Like a child facing her first day of kindergarten, my mother was terrified and panicked and didn't know what to expect. I, like a comforting parent, was calm and resolute and told her what would happen when she went in for her lumpectomy.

"Make sure they give you some anti-anxiety medication—Ativan, Valium, or something before they start the lymph node mapping," I advised.

I didn't tell her that I had nothing but a local anesthetic when they were sticking needles under my nipple. The kind doctor with a sexy French accent said, "We do not stick the needle *in* your nipple. We go *under* the nipple." Oh, yeah, that's *much* better!

I thought about this experience some more and said, "Mom, I'm going to call your doctor and ask her to give you a little something to take the edge off." That would be easier on the staff than picking my mother's fingernails out of the ceiling.

She was so nervous about her surgery, I immediately knew not to tell her that I had a positive lymph node. I was afraid it could be fatal and here's why:

My mom is a silent worrier. She's not real big on discussing her feelings. She feels deeply, but she doesn't emote, so she can come across as distant. As a child, I could tell when she was worried because she would fall asleep on the couch, and her mouth would be pinched in a frown. She would have two creases between her eyebrows deep enough to lay a toothpick down in each one. How someone could fall asleep without her face relaxing is still a mystery to me.

I knew if I told her about my positive lymph node she would take the worry into the operating room with her. There she would be completely sedated, but her anesthesiologist would look at her and say, "I don't know—look at those eyebrows. I'd better give her a little more." Overdose! Obviously I couldn't take that chance. I'd tell her about my node when she was out of surgery.

This was the moment where I felt the beginning of the role reversal between Mom and me. I had hints of it before: cleaning her house and cooking for her when she had gall bladder surgery; taking charge of the funeral when my grandmother died.

Not telling her about my lymph node was not the same as hiding the fact that I had slept with my college boyfriend—that was just plain self-preservation. No, this was different. For the first time in my life, she seemed small and vulnerable, and I wanted to protect her, to shield her from worry.

In the past, it always seemed as if we went right back to our old ways once everything got back to normal. But this time I knew there was no going back. I would always think about taking care of her from now on.

She was not going to grow stronger and more independent in the next ten years. The reverse was true.

Three

THE PLAN!

Dear Family and Friends,

Because I mentioned well-intentioned people saying "stupid, hurtful" things I received a mass of messages apologizing. It was not any of you, but actually someone who was visiting us.

He was going on about how cancer would force me to make changes in my life, I'd appreciate the small things, I would learn what's really important, and this was my wake-up call. These are golden words coming from someone who is speaking about their own experience. But it is instant crap when someone is telling you how you're going to feel.

He kind of forgot that I've been a chaplain for twenty years and that maybe I've learned something from my patients. He also said that *now* I would think about death, and I about fell over myself laughing. That is my favorite subject!

So I'm going to receive six months of CMF: a daily pill and a weekly intravenous infusion. They told me that CMF stands for Cytoxan, methotrexate and 5-fluorouracil. I know that it stands for: Crushed cockroach, Monkey vomit, and Floor sweepings. If that doesn't make cancer cells want to vacate my body, I don't know what will.

Of course, the chemo will put me into immediate menopause. This means that instead of taking the elevator and getting off on the menopause floor, I will be hurtling down the elevator shaft. Maybe it won't be so bad. I believe General Custer said something similar.

My plan (which I am holding lightly and gently) is to continue to work Tuesday, Wednesday, and Thursday. Then, on Thursday afternoon, instead of my usual cup of tea, I'll have my chemo. Just a slight change. And of course, I can still have tea.

Wes and I are truly doing great. My sister is here right now, and we are having a blast. She asked me what she could do for me. In a true test of sibling loyalty I said, "Scrub my shower." She was thrilled!

Physically I am doing well. My only complaint is about the colony of Mexican jumping beans living in my armpit, very close to my node scar. They seem to be having a fiesta, complete with Mariachi band, dancing at all hours. So it's constant twitching and I can't make it stop.

So that's the report. We are going to Wes's family reunion in Mexico for five days at the end of May. (Perhaps I can convince the jumping beans to return home.) My plan is to be back at work on June 14 and to get my first dose on the 16th.

I really miss you all so much. Thanks for your sweet cards and messages. And thanks for just being there.

Love and Hugs,
Debra

Wait, Wait Don't Tell Me

It wasn't as if our guest hadn't gone through his own very frightening health crisis, because he had. And perhaps people had spouted all kinds of advice to him, and therefore he thought that was the thing he should do. But it wasn't.

We were sitting out on our deck and Wes, having made a lovely dinner, was now in the house getting dessert. It was then that the sermon began.

"You're going to make some big changes in your life. This is really going to make you appreciate the small things. And—you'll start thinking about death." He let out a big sigh and stretched his arms over his head. "Yup, Deb. This is your wake-up call."

"Bullshit on that." I said it so venomously that he straightened up as if he might have to protect himself. "What in the hell do you think I've been doing for the past twenty years? You think I've learned nothing? My *wake-up* call? Are you saying I've been asleep all this time? I'm happy with my life and my job and the choices I've made. And the only change I'm going to make now is that I won't sit here and smile and nod when people like you say bullshit like that!"

He didn't have a chance to respond because Wes came out wearing a big smile and carrying a huge plate of strawberry short-cake. "Anyone for dessert?"

"Excuse me." I could not stay at the table. I went down into our basement, closed the door, and pressed my hot face against our washing machine. Yes, I was on narcotics for pain, but "*Bullshit on that*"? How uncreative. Why couldn't I have quoted scripture?

I should have quoted Job 12:2, 5: "What you know, I know also. I am not inferior to you. Oh, that you would be completely silent! Then you would be wise." Or Job 13:12! "Your memorable sayings are proverbs of ashes, your defenses are defenses of clay. Be silent, leave me alone, that I may speak."

Truly, I say unto you, that would have been perfect. Because when you are in the No Clue Zone (as we still were that day) you need people to help you speak, to help you sort out your feelings and give them a voice. You don't need platitudes or people telling you everything will be all right or telling you what your experience means.

But I could never have quoted Job because I am horrible at remembering Scripture, and I usually get it all wrong. I used to keep Psalm 33 memorized because years ago my hospice patients, especially the older ones, liked me to quote Psalms. But I've forgotten everything and standing in the basement with my head on the washer the only verse I could remember was, "Jesus wept." So I did.

I didn't need or want cancer to be my spiritual wake-up call. If I had to have one, well, why couldn't it come on a nice silent retreat? Or while reading poetry or Rumi? Or receiving Communion, or even something down-to-earth like pulling weeds?

While weeping on our washing machine, I noticed my rayon blouse that I had hung to dry. It was a stiff and wrinkled mess. My intention had been to save it from the trauma of dry cleaning so I hand washed it, but it turned out badly. I wasn't even sure I could salvage it.

Your intention was good, but the result was bad.

Mr. Martha Miyagi was talking to me in the basement. I wanted to crawl inside of our top-loading washer and close the lid. Whither can I go from thy spirit? It didn't matter because I could hear the Presence inside me suggesting that I judge our friend not on his behavior, but on his intention.

I do believe that intention matters. He would never want to hurt, offend, or upset me in any way. And what had made me so angry in the first place? Was I secretly afraid that I *had* been asleep?

I'd like to report I had the revelation that I couldn't salvage my blouse, but I could salvage my friendship, so I went back out on the deck. But that didn't happen. I did go back out on the deck, but only because I wanted the strawberry shortcake, damn it. I'm not proud of the fact that it took me a few days to let go of my resentment. I just kept reminding myself that he was doing the best he could. Everyone is doing the best they can. Plus, carrying around all that righteous indignation just didn't feel good. So first I had to stop talking about it because every time I told the story, I just fed my poor, wounded self. Then I could let it go.

And I pitched the rayon blouse.

Mail Bonding

While I'm on the subject of words helpful and unhelpful, let me share a few insights about e-mails. First of all, 99 percent of the messages I received were wonderful and met the following criteria: (1) acknowledgment that having cancer sucked, (2) personal compliments and encouragement, and (3) offers of support, either tangible or intangible. It was a bonus if the message was funny or contained humorous attachments like the video of the dog on the skateboard.

One of the first messages I received was from our friend Kevin who owns a beach house. It's a perfect example of tangible support.

> Hey, I'm sure that you've got plenty goin' on, but I jes
> wanted to throw something your way. If, after surgery,
> or whenever, you'd like to just get away (while folks
> always mean well, the sheer volume of calls, visitors,
> even flower deliveries to the front door can be a pain),

we'd love to offer up our island house for some "rehab" as needed. You'd be secluded as hell, just the two of you, the water, the whales, the eagles, and Mother Nature. Ooh-la-la! Holler anytime, for anything.

His message was simple, caring, and straightforward—here's what I can offer you and call for anything.

The one from my boss still makes me weep because I find it so touching. Of course, he *is* a trained chaplain.

> I hope you are staying on top of the pain with pain meds and that each day is better. I have heard that one of the patients commented how touched she was by your phone call. You are incredible. I am grateful for how much your relationships with patients mean to you (and to them). I write this while also hoping you will take very good care of yourself. You are so important to me, as well as to all of us. I suspect this is much tougher than you are telling. My heart and prayers are with you. May your heart be comforted in all the areas that it hurts and worries; may your wounds heal thoroughly and timely; may you know invigorating health; may you know how loved you are; may the love of your life, Wes, know peace, comfort, and strength; may you celebrate with great joy each healing phase.
> Missing you,
> Stephen

What I love about his message is that it is personal (he knows that Wes is the love of my life, and that I tend to minimize things), complimentary (he calls me 'incredible'), and caring (may your wounds heal thoroughly).

I was forced to leave work in an untimely manner, and as I sat home popping pain pills, I knew that life at the SCCA was going on as usual. I wondered if anyone missed me. It's a childish fear born out of insecurity, but as I said before, one tends to regress with a serious illness. But that's why the line, "You are so important to me as well as to all of us," made me cry. It was just what I needed to hear, that I wasn't forgotten and that I was missed.

During this regressive period, I also developed a craving (more than usual) for compliments and praise. I wasn't at work, where I got a sense of personal gratification every day. The only thing I was doing while I was home was writing updates. So when I received this message from my friend Teresa, I lapped it up.

> So I was sitting here (okay, sprawled) contemplating eating the three Häagen-Dazs ice cream bars in the freezer, when I decided to check on my e-mail. To my delight, Debra, your e-mail was shining in my inbox. Yes, shining. All the other pathetic little messages hung their fonts in shame. How, after major surgery no less, can you manage to write something so warm, clever, and inspiring? Hell, I had a difficult conference call, and I'm ready to go for a "lactose overdose" courtesy of Vanilla Almond on a Stick. I apparently have to teach you how to whine and complain. Once you master that, I'll introduce you to my friends in the freezer—Ben and Jerry. Thanks so much for the update. I will continue to keep you and Wes in my prayers.

Even if she hadn't praised my writing, her message was hilarious. But she didn't kill herself trying to be funny.

I say write as if you are actually talking to the person—like this message from my friend Michele whose husband was dealing with prostate cancer:

> Listen baby,
> It is a shitty card to be dealt no matter how you go at it. And that Wes, I am smokin' up prayers for that boy. I think I know his anxiety and fear. But there are

a cascade of blessings amidst a shit-load of pain, fear, suffering, and dread. I have found it to have changed basically everything. Too much to talk about. Through our experience, Chuck and I are closer than ever, closer to our true selves, able to pray together and help each other in ways we couldn't have imagined. I love you both, even from a distance of space and time. We are holding you close.

She acknowledges the pain of diagnosis and surgery, etc., shares that she got through it, points out that there are blessings to be found, and then gives an example about being closer to her husband. She tells me she loves us and is praying for us. This is huge. You cannot underestimate the power of telling people that you love them and pray for them.

She talks a little bit about Chuck, but she doesn't go on and on, and believe me she could have because they had their own crappy cancer circus going on. She would be an excellent chaplain because she shares about herself from her heart, but keeps the focus on the other person.

Sending a Bible verse or two about how God is always present or how we can't be separated from the love of God is nice. But nix the pages of scripture in the King James filled with verses about our "present sufferings"; the creation and the spirit groaning (all I could think was, "Where are the pain meds?"); and trouble, hardship, persecution, famine, nakedness, danger, and swords. Did I mention glorification and justification and how we are considered as sheep to be slaughtered? When you're fresh out of surgery, you're already feeling a little slaughtered. The last image you want to carry around in your mind is a bloody sheep.

My best friend from junior high sent me a wonderful message with a list of well-known women who have been breast cancer survivors for years. This was encouraging. If you know women who have died of breast cancer—just keep that to yourself.

Finally, an e-mail message that just made me smile. It's from a young man whose wedding I officiated.

> A. You inspire the crap out of me.
> B. You are an amazing writer.
> C. You touch me with your experiences and make me realize that tough stuff is, not only doable, but required for a full life. Thanks for reminding me. Keep on truckin' Rev. You are truly one in a million.
> Much love,
> Ian Walker

So in case you get constipated, keep reading, and I'll inspire the crap out of you.

Missing the Point

I was able to check my work e-mail from home, and I was sad to receive a message that one of my favorite patients, Ted Christos, had died. He was a seventy-five-year-old Greek Orthodox man. We would get into long conversations about the Orthodox liturgy and why they didn't ordain women. "It's just wrong," he said. I didn't pursue that line of conversation because I knew it would be fruitless.

But he was thrilled that I had taken several classes with a Greek Orthodox priest, and the classes were actually held in an Orthodox church. He was even more thrilled to find out that I had done a weekend retreat with the church and learned how to paint an icon. I brought it in for him to see. It was of Christ the teacher where Jesus is holding a book in one hand and holding up the other in a blessing pose. Ted liked it very much but had one criticism.

"Good, but the eyes of Jesus are too big."

"The eyes of Jesus—what a great title for a book!"

He laughed and then said, "I'm writing a book."

"You are? What's it about?"

He told me how he was writing a children's book for his granddaughter.

"Maybe you would look at it? Help me get it published?"

"Sure!" I said. I was excited. Maybe it could be published before he died. His prognosis was not good. He had metastatic gastric cancer. The next week he brought in a fifty-page manuscript.

"It's about a crow," he said thrusting an envelope at me. A crow—how cute! I couldn't wait to read it.

That night I opened it up and began reading. It began with a crow flying onto the bedroom windowsill of a young girl (presumably his granddaughter) as she is staring out the window and not doing her homework.

I got out my red pen. That was my fatal mistake. I spent over two hours correcting spelling and grammar and pointing out erratic change in verb tense. The young girl was speaking like a college student. The crow was getting annoying. The whole thing was preachy, and a lot of it was boring. But I could help him. I made arrows to indicate paragraph moves and wrote suggestions and questions in the margins. I cut out entire paragraphs. I sat back satisfied. I couldn't wait to see him.

He returned the following week for his chemo. I sat on the rolling stool next to his wheelchair and began my critique. I got to about page five and was saying, "See, all of a sudden you have the crow speaking with a British accent and using all these Cockney expressions—" He hadn't said anything so I turned to him. The look on his face was hatred, revulsion, loathing, disgust.

"Ted! What?"

He snatched the manuscript out of my hands and said, "I'm tired and want to take a little nap now. Thank you."

I felt as if someone had just dropped an anvil on my head. How could I have been so stupid? He didn't want criticism, he wanted approval. He never again spoke to me after that day. Every time I peeked in his room, he would pretend he was sleeping.

I sent him a little card apologizing and told him I missed talking with him. He didn't care.

I had wanted to do something uplifting for him, and it was as if I had crushed him.

Family Herstory

My sister, Lynie, was supposed to be here for my surgery, but the day before she was to fly out, her son had appendicitis. When that happened we started thinking maybe there *was* a plague upon our house, what with my mom and me and then my nephew. But as I've said before, shit happens.

Lynie is two years younger than me and up until two weeks before, had no family history of breast cancer. Now suddenly she had a major one. My mom and Lynie and I are all members of the Dense Breast Society, also known as the Sack of Rocks Club. Our mammograms are hard to read. We have cysts and benign fibrous tumors. I started getting yearly mammograms in my thirties because I had so many lumps.

Lynie is very calm about these things and assured me that as soon as she got home she was going to talk to her doctor about her new history. I was happy about this since I felt this irrational guilt about providing her a risk factor for breast cancer.

I wanted my sister with me, because, well, she's my sister. Who I am is tied up in our shared history, especially the history of our bodies. I knew she had a heart murmur when she was a toddler. She knew I had a big tumor when I was a little baby. I was the first person she told when she started her period. She was the only person I told when I sunburned my breasts by lying topless at the beach.

It turned out that it was just as well that she came a couple weeks after my surgery, because by that time, I was a little more mobile. I was already up to walking three miles a day, and I really wanted her to meet Max.

I don't want to be coy or cute about this, so right up front I want you to know that Max is a dog—a wheat-colored cairn terrier—Toto from *The Wizard of Oz*.

Before I started chemo, I went to see a naturopath who told me that if I walked briskly for forty-five minutes a day, it would help me get through chemotherapy. It was on my first brisk walk that I met Max.

The woman holding his leash that day was walking toward Wes and me. Max saw us and leaped ecstatically toward us, his leash making a diagonal line across the street. He looked up at me with a look that said, "At last! I've found you! Yes, you. You're the one I've been waiting for." I carefully bent down to pet him and he gave my face a thorough licking.

I said to the woman, "Oh, my God, I love him."

"Really?" she asked, laughing. "Do you want him?"

My eyes widened. "Yes!" Wes looked shocked and later told me he thought it was the pain meds talking.

It turned out that Max lived across the street from this woman, Amy. She walked him every day because his owner never did. "He is married with two small children. Max is out in the front yard twenty-four/seven, and the guy just doesn't have time for him."

I was horrified. Why would anyone keep this fabulous dog outside all the time? Why not just get a goat?

"You can go over and play with him any time," Amy said. "That's what everyone in the neighborhood does. He's always out there. I'll ask his owner if he wants to give him away."

So Max was the reason that I would haul myself out of bed every morning for my walk. I would call out his name from three houses down and then watch his head go up and down behind the fence as if he were on a pogo stick.

I mostly threw a tennis ball for him. Although I wanted to, I didn't get too affectionate with him. I was healing from my surgery, and the thought of him jumping on my incision made my skin crawl.

Lynie is something of a dog expert, so as soon as she dropped her bags, I suggested we go for a brisk walk—to meet Max.

Of course she loved him. She played with him, threw the ball, scratched his belly, watched him run around, and then said, "I don't think you would be running into any big problems with this little dog."

The sisterly seal of approval. I was thrilled. Now I just had to wait for Amy to ask Max's owner if he wanted to give him away.

The next day Lynie, Wes, and I went to my first appointment with my oncologist. She is very smart, talks very fast, and loves, loves, loves statistics. If she told the story of the three bears it would go something like this:

"Some time between the years 1200 and 1400, a female between the ages of 8 and 11 with a probable mortality rate of 43 percent, was walking through a forest, which was 74 percent old growth timber, 11 percent new growth, and 15 percent undetermined, when she came upon a 300-square-foot cottage, which in the price range of that time was worth approximately one year's crop of wheat and a cow. Upon seeing three bowls on the table of varying sizes, she had a 33⅓ percent chance of finding one that she would deem suitable for her purposes, where N=3, the p value is less than .01, with a mean of 2.64."

You can see she must have no problem putting her son to sleep.

So she gave us all the information and all the statistics. And like a mother bird that eats, digests, then throws-up for her chicks, Wes took in the data and fed it back to me in a palatable form.

The choice was basically no chemo and tamoxifen, or, to get a few more percentage points of insurance against recurrence, I could have chemo plus tamoxifen. My rationale for choosing chemo was that I didn't want to have a recurrence five years down the line and say, "Dagnabit! I should have done the chemo." But of course I'd never say, "Dagnabit."

"And you won't lose all your hair, but you'll lose some."

Ah, yes, the hair. That's one of the first things people asked me about when I told them I had breast cancer.

"Will you lose your hair?"

Some people just assumed I would. "There goes the hair," an acquaintance said, trying to be light and funny. Her hair was fine and thin and split on the ends.

I looked at her and thought, "You'd love for me to lose my hair." As you can see, cancer was not always bringing out the best in me.

I mean, it's true, especially for women, that when you lose your hair, you lose part of your identity. It seems unfair that on top of getting cancer you lose your hair. However, like losing your breasts, for some women it's a bigger deal than for others.

But the thing is, it's not really about the hair. It's really about death. People die from cancer all the time. But it's so impolite to say, "Will you lose your life?" It's much easier to ask about the hair.

Because if you don't lose your hair, you can almost pretend that you don't have cancer. Sure, you may be tired and nauseated. Your surgery site may hurt. You may have sores in your mouth. Your fingernails may be falling off and getting infected. But these are not things that people notice immediately or at all.

No one can look at you and say, "Chemo patient." And if you have a sure hand with makeup, you can look downright healthy if you haven't lost your hair.

But if you go bald, you are marked. You can't pretend that everything is normal and that you don't think about death. It's hard for others to pretend they don't think about death when they look at you.

Your bald head shoves death in their faces. And most people really hate thinking about dying. So they struggle to ask the right questions. Is asking, "What's your prognosis?" too nosey? The answer to that could just lead to more awkwardness. It's safer to talk about hair.

But here's the good thing about losing your hair: you *can't* pretend that everything is normal. One woman who had just lost her hair to chemo said to me, "I had chemo for three years and never lost my hair. My family acted as if nothing was wrong. Where are my jeans? Did you call the travel agent? What's for dinner? But now, my God, they're freaking out and they're falling over themselves to help me."

Another patient told me that she wished she *had* lost her hair so everyone would stop saying how good she looked. She wanted to scream, "But I feel crappy! The outside doesn't match the inside!" But that's often how it is for healthy people, too. You can look great and be miserable.

No, it's not about the hair, but people want to make it about the hair because it's so hard to listen to someone talk about fear and pain and grief. It's the same reason my friend went on with his platitudes—it was too hard for him to listen to me. It might even cause him to feel his own painful emotions. But if you can listen to someone talk about those feelings, then when you do talk about the hair, it will really be about the hair.

That was one of the great things about having Lynie around: I could talk to her about anything. Well, almost anything. The one thing we couldn't talk about was her estrangement from my parents. I'm not even sure now what the original dispute was about, but there were hurt feelings on both sides. Like many things of this nature, the longer it goes on, the longer it goes on. It had been going on for sixteen years. But I come from a long line of grudge bearers on the hotheaded Spanish side of my family: fathers and mothers, sons and daughters, brothers and sisters who don't speak to one another. Changing allegiances. Shifting alliances. I can't even guess at the wounds and pain that they all carry.

Over the years, I was determined not to edit my conversation with either my sister or my parents. So I would cheerfully report to my parents about a visit with Lynie and tell Lynie about visiting Mom and Dad.

These comments were met with what I sensed was strained enthusiasm or forced neutrality. Over the years, I had to give up my desire for them to reconcile. I gave it up approximately six hundred times. Each time I got a little better at letting go. But now I had cancer and like a herpes virus that lies dormant and is suddenly activated, the desire came back with a vengeance.

I thought perhaps both mom and I getting cancer would remind everyone that life is too short, and let's just be a loving family. Forgive and forget! Or remember and reconcile! For God's sake, it's your child! It's your parents! I had prayed about this, seeing them all surrounded by Light—merciful, forgiving, loving Light. What I probably should have done was see myself surrounded by Light—detached, non-judgmental, trusting Light.

Here is a little-talked-about danger with cancer (as if it's not dangerous enough): because you are forced to think hard about your own life, you think everyone else should, too. You think they should get their shit together—according to your agenda. There is a temptation to say, "Hey! I have *cancer*, listen unto me."

It's a form of emotional manipulation and it's dangerous. Cancer does not give you immediate wisdom, insight, and understanding. If you do gain any wisdom, insight, or understanding, it's not because of the cancer per se, but because the cancer has forced you to do your inner work.

Your having cancer also does not suddenly wake up everyone else. If they weren't listening to you before, they're not going to listen to you now. Maybe they will if it looks like you going to die very soon. Even then, they'll probably all be in denial about that or say that you're overmedicated or even demented. Unless they ask you for your opinion on some long-standing issue, it's better to just shut up. So I didn't talk to Lynie about any of this—for now. But it was heavy on my heart.

After the oncologist appointment, Lynie, Wes, and I went to Blue C Sushi for dinner. This is the kind of place where different kinds of sushi go by on a conveyor belt and you grab what you want. We were a bit overwhelmed with information, and I was feeling sober, serious, and life-threatened. So this was the perfect place to go, because there's something goofy and uplifting about watching your dinner go by on a little train. It pulls you out of yourself—you can't be self-absorbed and snag the spider maki at the same time.

The place was hopping because it's fairly cheap and close to the university. I looked around at people laughing, drinking, eating and thought, "No matter what happens to me, life goes on. At some point I'm going to die, and every single person in this place is going to die." This may sound morbid, but I had just eaten the *uni*, the sea urchin, which does look like decomposing flesh. Thoughts of death came easily.

I found that thought, "everyone dies," comforting. It was comforting in the same way that when I saw young women and felt envious or nostalgic for, say firm skin and no cellulite, I'd think, "You will be my age some day. God willing."

I thought, "The battle with the body will never be won. It's best to accept it, and just carry on." I felt quite British when thinking this, stiff upper lip and all—as opposed to injected upper lip.

As I mentioned before, friends and family really wanted to help. So Lynie truly was thrilled to vacuum, scrub my shower, and wash dishes. I missed vacuuming. It's the thing I do when I don't know what to do with myself or when I'm upset or confused. I love the instant gratification. Visible dust balls? Gone. Crumbs on the floor? Gone. Tracked in pine needles? Gone. If only life were that easy. Twenty pounds overweight? Gone. Annoying coworker? Gone. Invasive cancer? Gone.

Anyway, when you're looking at recuperating from surgery and six months of chemotherapy, the immediate satisfaction of vacuuming is quite enticing. But I had been warned that next to making beds, vacuuming was one of the worst possible things to do when recovering from a mastectomy. So I lay on the couch and watched enviously as Lynie vacuumed the entire house.

I did not lie on the couch the whole time she was in town. We did go out. I couldn't drive, so she drove us to the mall where I looked for a particular candle with a smell that made me feel cheerful and loved and happy. All that from a scented candle! I had been given the candle for my birthday and burned it all the way down. In the candle store we were like crazed beagles madly sniffing everything on display.

"Found it!" I barked after ten minutes of sniffing. The scent was "Citrus and Sage." I wanted to buy everything in the store that carried this scent, and believe me they had infusers, candles, sprays, sachets, and I think I saw scented tennis balls. I carried the candle over to Lynie and waved it under her nose.

"Don't you just love it?" I asked. "I don't know why I love it so much. I just do!"

She took one sniff and said, "It smells like Wes."

"What?" I sniffed again and realized, that, oh, my God, yes, it smelled just like his aftershave.

"I guess that means you like having him around."

She was absolutely right.

Learn, Baby, Learn

Recuperating from my surgery gave me plenty of time to think about my patients. Perhaps it was because Wes and I were so happy together that it especially pained me when a patient in a healthy, happy relationship did poorly. I had been following Jason for a couple years. He and Linda had been married for ten and had two little boys. The chemotherapy he received for his leukemia didn't work. There were only so many tricks up his oncologist's sleeve, and the stem cell transplant was the last one. It didn't work.

So there he had been, on a ventilator in the ICU with no hope of coming off of it. This happened a few months before my diagnosis, before I really understood how much suffering a partner goes through. But I did understand that this was the most agonizing decision of Linda's life—she decided to turn it off. She had reached a place of peace and calm about it. She asked me to pray and stay with her as they took Jason off the ventilator. Linda and I were about to enter Jason's room, when the surgical resident suddenly appeared.

He planted himself directly in front of her. "Linda," he said. "I'm so sorry about Jason. I did everything I could. But I feel like such a failure. We went into his chest twice, and I don't think we could go in again. But I feel like a quitter. It's so terrible."

Linda looked stunned during this declaration, but she gently touched his arm and said, "It's okay. It's not your fault. You did everything you could."

He hung his head. "Well, I know. You're right. But I still feel like a failure."

After he left, Linda asked me, "What was I supposed to say to him?"

I shook my head. "I can't believe it! Your husband is about to die, and he's asking you to reassure him that he's a good doctor."

This experience haunted me for days. I was righteously indignant! I wanted to tell that surgeon to park his ego when it came to patient care. If I didn't tell him, who knew how much more damage he would do?

I can be a real jerk about stuff like this and I, Super Chaplain Defender of Patients, wanted to go in on my white horse, draw my sword, and take that doctor down. I knew that would be wrong, but I didn't know exactly what I *should* do.

My boss told me to forget about it. "He'll never listen to you."

Wes said, "Page him through the hospital operator and talk to him on the phone."

That would be the option that required the most courage on my part. I'd need a big horse, an enormous sword, and lots of armor. As I was pondering these options, a memory from my own internship twenty years ago came back to me.

A patient's wife had asked me if my parents liked Wes, who was my fiancé at the time. "Oh, yes. It's not like he's an ex-con or anything," I had answered.

On my next visit to this patient, his wife pulled me aside and had gently said, "My husband is an ex-convict. But he's paid his dues and he's a wonderful man. I just wanted you to know that."

I died a thousand deaths right there, but it was a big learning moment for me. She not only taught me about thinking before I speak, but she did so in a kind and compassionate way. And so I decided to talk to the doctor—no horse, no sword, and no armor.

A surgical nurse returned my page. "We're just about to go into surgery, he's scrubbed in now, he'll be in surgery all day," she said. "Oh—wait a minute—it looks like we're waiting for a pathology report to come in before we can operate. So you *can* talk to him. Hold on."

I told him who I was and he remembered the situation.

"I know that was a really hard case for you," I said. "I just wanted to check in with you and see how you're doing."

"Oh, yeah," he said. "I felt so bad about that case. I did everything I could. It was so hard. I felt horrible." His voice sounded kind of echoey, and I figured it must be the acoustics in the OR.

"I know. I just want to make sure you know that his death had nothing to do with your skill as a surgeon. His death was not your failure and though it's normal to feel like a failure at a time like that, you might not want to share those feelings with a family member. Maybe talk with a colleague or one of us chaplains."

"I don't think I said 'failure,'" he said sharply. I was silent.

"I guess I did say failure. Did his wife say something?"

"Well, yes, she did. You know, this isn't a criticism. It's just feedback to help you be a better doctor."

Now he was silent. "I guess it sort of took her out of the moment," he finally said.

"Yes."

We ended our conversation with me saying I hoped to see him again and he mumbled something back.

I went home that night and told Wes the whole story.

"You know," he said. "When you're all scrubbed in for surgery, they don't just hand you the phone. They put you on speakerphone."

"Speakerphone?!" I gasped.

I was so glad I got down off my horse and was kind to him. Because really, all of us are doing the best we can.

Chemopause

I am vain. As a high school freshman, I loved being mistaken for a senior. As a fifty-year-old woman, I loved being told I looked forty. But I knew what happened when your estrogen was yanked away. Because my tumor was estrogen- and progesterone-receptor positive (ER+, PR+), I could not take any replacement estrogen. *Au contraire!* The big "E" had to be banished forever and that meant menopause.

I had seen patients go into immediate menopause, and it's intense. No gradual slide into warm flashes and then hot flashes. It was more like a nuclear bomb going off. I had no problem with menopause itself, but I hated that it was forced upon me before my time. That just annoyed me to no end.

As if that weren't bad enough, my mother was reminding me what happened when her estrogen shut down. "Dry skin. Dry hair. *Everything* gets dry. And suddenly you have wrinkles! It's hell getting old."

But like mine, her tumor was ER+, PR+, and she couldn't have any estrogen either. So she had to stop taking her replacement estrogen, and now she was having hot flashes all over again. There *was* a plague upon our house.

So I hated that I would be aging from chemo. I hated that all my exercise, good eating habits, and Crème de la Mer couldn't stop what chemopause would do. The only way I could get over this was to check my breathing. In-breath or out-breath? Stay in the body, stay in the present—then I was okay. But I still wished it wasn't forced on me.

That's a control issue and the way to deal with that is to practice letting go.

Sometimes the Divine sounded more Martha Stewart than Mr. Miyagi. I knew that I suffered only when I wanted what I couldn't have. I had to stop wanting not to age, not to be in menopause. And on that day I cancelled my subscription to my favorite beauty magazine, *Allure*. It just made me want what I couldn't have.

Making a Plan and Checking It Twice

My case manager told me that many people on CMF are able to continue working. That seemed like the thing for me to do. For one thing, it's really easy to get self-absorbed when you have cancer. The whole treatment process encourages that because you're getting a weekly blood test, your nurse is asking you questions, and everyone seems more concerned than usual about you. I didn't need any encouragement to be self-absorbed. Seeing patients, being with staff, and focusing on others would balance things out.

My boss understood this since many times in the past I had said, "I'm feeling cranky. I need to see a patient." Whenever I had been in a bad mood in the past, I would visit a patient and always feel better. It wasn't that I needed to see someone in worse shape than I was, it was something about the interaction, the communication, the feeling that I was doing and being exactly what I was supposed to. I knew working would be therapeutic for me.

I could also go back to work because I didn't have anyone depending on me for physical care. Wes was healthy, we have no kids, and our beloved dog died a few years back.

Getting a cancer diagnosis when you have children at home is a whole different ball game. In fact, it's not a ball game at all, but more like a wrestling match. You are wrestling with the fact that you feel like crap, but the kids still need their diapers changed or lunches packed, or must be schlepped off to soccer or diving practice. If you have a partner, he or she still needs affection and attention. But when fatigue and nausea have a chokehold on you, it's hard to think of anything else.

I thought I could manage to work my usual three days a week. However, I was going to hold that plan lightly and gently because I knew everyone reacted to chemo differently. But I was starting out from a strong place—I had been training for a triathlon when I was diagnosed. I hoped that being in good shape would serve me well the next six months.

Yeah, I was in perfect health—except for the cancer.

Death Doesn't Take a Holiday

Just because I was off work recovering from surgery didn't mean my patients were on hold. They continued to recover or decline.

Eleanor continued to decline and had been on hospice for two months. She was sixty years old and from New York. She and her husband Harvey had that east coast way of talking that makes you feel as if they're arguing with you. She was sharp and edgy and funny and angry.

Harvey had been coming in to see me for counseling. Well, it wasn't really counseling. I hardly said a word because Harvey would rave non-stop for about forty-five minutes and then spend about five minutes thanking me profusely and telling me how much better he felt.

I had told Harvey that I would be off for a few weeks. "Oh, no problem, that's fine, I'm fine, we'll be fine, we have friends."

But the chaplain covering for me called me and said that he had left several voice mail messages for me. "He sounded distressed," she said.

So I called him and resigned myself to a forty-five minute phone call. But I was wrong. He didn't want to talk.

"Debra," he said, "Can you come over? It's happening. Eleanor is dying. She seems upset. She's struggling. She's mumbling. She's picking at the sheets. This is terrible! This is just horrible!" Pause. "What is it, my darling? Are you waking up? I'm talking to Debra." I could hear voices in the background.

"Who's there with you, Harvey?"

"The hospice team: her nurse, the social worker, the chaplain. But if you could come, Debra, I think Eleanor will settle down. Eleanor, do you want Debra to come? Hmm?" Pause. "Eleanor isn't responding, but I thought you could say something to give her some peace."

Some people have amazing transformations before they die. One of my hospice patients changed so much that his ex-wife remarried him. "He became the man I knew was in there when I married him," she said to me. "He lost his real self for many years, but he found it again. I was happy to love him and care for him as he died."

This doesn't happen often. Many people die the way they live. Eleanor was not someone who would die gently. She never did anything gently.

"Harvey," I replied, "There is nothing that I can say that will give Eleanor peace. She is doing this her way. Not everybody has a peaceful death." I didn't even mention that I was recovering from surgery because that wasn't the reason I refused to come. I could hear Harvey crying, and all the little pleaser and guilt bells were ringing in my head. I had to put my hand over my mouth to stop myself from saying anything else.

"Okay," he said. "I've got lots of support here. But she's dying!"

"I know, Harvey. I'll keep you both in my prayers."

We hung up and I sat right down, closed my eyes, and visualized them all surrounded by the Light. I held this for a long time.

I've been with lots of people as they've died. It's like watching a candle go out: the flame flickers ferociously because the wax is gone, then flickers more gently, then *poof!* it's out. For a moment there remains that glowing wick and you think, it's still here! It's going to burn again! But then the glow fades to black and a thin stream of white smoke rises up. Then you know, for sure, at last, the flame is gone. Nothing left but the candle stub, still warm. And you can see so clearly that the candle is not the flame. It is not the candle that gives light and warmth, but the flame. But of course, where is the flame without the candle?

When I opened my eyes I started to wonder about my own death. Would I go gently? Or would I be cracking jokes and demanding See's Candies? Would I get out of my body with everyone there or would I sneak out when I was alone?

How would I be in a fatal car crash? I really hoped I wouldn't say, "Oh shit," because that is just so *common.* That's what most airplane pilots say as they're going down. How about "Hell yeah!"

What about a stabbing? As the life ebbed out of me would I be fumbling for my lipstick? I'd probably try to crawl somewhere that could be easily cleaned, my mother's voice echoing through my head, "Don't eat in the living room!"

I really want to be thinking some good thoughts like, "Woo-hoo! Whatta ride!" or "What's next?" or "Holy-Jesus-God-and-All-the-Saints, Buddha, Allah, here I come!"

Or maybe just a simple, "Thank you."

Four

THE PORT REPORT

Dearest Family and Friends,

I thought I'd wait until I had my port-a-cath placed to send an update. The port is a catheter, which they stuck under the skin on my chest. It is about the size of a woman's Timex watch. It is attached to a line that runs into a big vein in my chest area. I will receive my chemo directly through the port and won't have to be stuck in the arm every week to put a line in for the infusion.

I had my port placed on Thursday. I knew something was amiss when I woke up and the resident said in a falsely cheery voice, "Doesn't she look great? She looks like she just came back from the spa!"

I immediately thought, "Nice try—what's wrong?"

It turns out that after two hours of digging, prodding, and general horsing around, they could not get the line into my subclavian vein, so yes, they went for the jugular! I'll tell you right now, no amount of cherry flavored oxycodone would make me go through that again.

Because I am returning to work this Tuesday, and the steri-strips on my neck will still be in place, I foresee two types of jokes coming at me: (1) vampire jokes, and (2) hickey jokes. You have my permission to knock yourselves out.

Replacement Parts Department: I had a saline implant/tissue expander put in at the time of my mastectomy. This is where they cut through my pectoralis muscle, made a little pocket, and shoved—excuse me—*placed* a partially filled implant in the pocket and sewed me back up. There is then a port sticking out the side of my breast that looks just like the thingy through which you blow up a child's wading pool. Except that this is under my skin. E-e-w-w.

Then, my masochistic, I mean, *altruistic* plastic surgeon filled it once a week. This did not hurt—at first. But the next forty-eight hours had me tearing out my hair and confessing to all sorts of crimes that I did not commit. Anything to stop the pain. Then I was fine.

I think I could have been done with one filling, but my surgeon did two. Our conversation went like this:

Me: "Wow! I think it's too big!"

Doctor: "No, no—it's still swollen."

Me: "Is this a guy thing?"

Doctor: "No, no. Come back in a month and if it's too big, I'll take some out."

Me: "If it's still this big in a month, I'm gonna come back and put a port-a-cath in your jugular!"

He fainted.

So for my male friends: You get one look, two at the most. It is the right side. It's no big deal, and I mean that literally. Then you can go back to admiring my intellect and wit.

Finally, some have suggested that perhaps I am in denial because they think I'm way too cheerful about all of this. Here is what I have to say about that: I have seen women half my age come in with breast cancer at twice my stage. So I have a nice correction to my perspective. It doesn't mean I have not been deeply annoyed by much of this.

The grief it has caused my family and friends has been hard to bear. It's been hard to watch Wes run himself ragged doing everything. When I came home from the port placement they said, "Don't lift anything heavier than oxycodone with your left arm." And I still don't have full function in my right arm. So that meant I was an armless, constipated stoner for two days. I hated that. Wes was actually fine, so I decided to simply get over it.

Cancer has not made me start to think about the big issues. You know that the purpose of life, spirituality, dying, and death are all things I've been yakking about for years. So it's like, "*Oy vey*. Again with the meaning of life?"

I know there is Something Bigger than all of us that connects us to one another in a wonderful and mysterious way. It is up to me to find meaning in this experience. The hero/heroine's journey is never about simply slaying the dragon. The task within the task is to slay the dragon while finding meaning, gaining wisdom, and doing it with some grace and charm. I figure if I can go through cancer treatment without losing my inner joy, and with some measure of compassion and good humor, it is better for all of us.

The sermon is now over. Will the ushers please come forward? We will receive the morning offering.

My mom is doing great. She had a lumpectomy and her nodes were clear. She is back to gardening and complaining about her hairdresser—a sure sign of recovery.

I can't thank you enough for your flowers, cards, e-mails, prayers, and good thoughts. Just before my diagnosis, I was given a gorgeous temporary office. Last week they took it back—an officectomy—another painful procedure. It's okay— I loved every moment in that beautiful office because I knew it was temporary. Just like life.

Much Love and Hugs,
Debra

Reconstruction

Many women have told me that their breasts are important to their sexual identity. One woman told me she hated to give up the breasts that fed her babies. Another woman said she would miss propping up her reading on her "shelf" as she called it.

The most I could prop up on my breasts were toast crumbs, so I was not grieving the loss of my breast like many women do. But there was that question of, "What goes there now?"

Because I am basically lazy and dislike hassle, the thought of putting a prosthesis in my bra did not appeal to me. I also had the happy problem of not having enough fat on my belly for one of the flap procedures. That was okay with me since I didn't relish the thought of an eight-hour surgery and then waking up in the ICU.

I wanted to be able to put on my clothes or slip into a swimsuit and go. Wes said his love for me was not dependent on me having breasts, or "time bombs," as he now referred to them. "Whatever you choose is fine by me," he said. So the implant seemed like the easiest thing to do.

It was easy but painful. My implant was both an expander and an implant at the same time. Once it was the correct size, my plastic surgeon removed the port from the implant, and it self-sealed. This saved me from having to get another surgery. He said after each filling I might feel some discomfort.

Perhaps we need a clarification on the word "discomfort." The dictionary definition is "very mild pain." To me "very mild pain" is a paper cut, hitting your funny bone, or getting a sliver in your finger.

The implant filling was more along the lines of slamming your hand in the car door or being eaten by a wild animal. He was correct, however, that I did not feel "discomfort" immediately. It took about an hour before I felt like shrieking. I am told it is not like this for everyone, and to that I can only shout, "Thank ya, Jesus!"

At the final filling my plastic surgeon, the resident, and my husband were all looking critically at my boobs. Did they match? How much would the swelling go down? Do not think this bothered me in the least. I was actually yawning. By that point, so many people had looked at my breasts I could have walked topless into the anniversary sale at Nordstrom and not blinked an eye.

So there was something there to fill a bra, but it was not the same shape as my real breast. My real one is more cone-shaped, like a miniature Mt. Rainier except without the snow and volcanic peak. The implant was more like half a baseball. I would have said half an orange, but I hate how fruit terms apply to women and sporting equipment terms apply to men.

I was not grieving the loss of my breast, but I was grieving the loss of ease with my body. My implant was uncomfortable all the time. I thought twice about reaching for things with my right hand. Never did I realize how much I used my pectoral muscles. I could hardly do anything that required pressure from my right hand. This meant not only could I not chop, but also I couldn't wash my face, scrub the sink, or applaud. I couldn't believe that last one.

But then, how many opportunities would you think I'd have to clap? Lots. That's the thing with cancer—the plans you made before your diagnosis are still in place. Some of them you have to cancel, but others you can keep. Having cancer does not mean your whole life stops. You simply adjust or modify your plans.

For example, Wes cancelled his teaching trips to Montana and Alaska so he could be with me for my surgery. That was a no-brainer. But on the calendar we had theatre plans about two weeks after my surgery. My friend, Robyn, wrote and starred in the play *Gravity*, and her husband Steve directed it. Wes and I both really wanted to see it. So dressed in my black warm-up suit (the one for formal occasions) and armed with my bottle of oxycodone, we went. That is where I first noticed I couldn't clap properly.

So I adopted this way of clapping my left hand against my right palm as it lay in my lap. It looked so affected, as if I were in some British movie saying, "Yes, quite so. Indeed." The audience was enthusiastic. I didn't want them to think my restrained clapping meant I didn't like the play. I also had just enough oxycodone on board to feel a little loose, so as I clapped like the Queen of England, I yelled, "Yay! Yay! Yay!"

I was glad we went to the play because I got out of the house and back into the outside world. It was also one of Mr. Martha Miyagi's most novel ways of speaking to me. The most unusual thing about the production (besides the trapeze work and the shower of shoes at the end) was the stage itself.

Imagine a perfectly square platform balanced on top of a pyramid. So it turned, tilted, and tipped whenever anyone moved on it. Unless Robyn was standing right in the middle of it, she would fall off. Unless she was centered she would go down. Everyone who came onto the stage changed the balance of things, and she would have to adjust her position. At one point she was hanging on by her fingernails.

Isn't that just the perfect description of having cancer? Everyone and everything—people, medical tests, side effects—change the balance of your life and you have to adjust. Sometimes you feel as if you are hanging on by your fingernails. But all of it is manageable if you *stay centered.*

Quite so. Indeed.

You're Not Dead Yet

My first week back at work there was no gradual re-entry, no slowly walking down the steps into the shallow end of the pool.

No, it was right off the high dive the moment I came in. I received a page that a patient needed to see me immediately.

The case manager explained the situation: the patient, Robert, whose initial stem-cell transplant failed, was hoping to get his lymphoma into remission to receive another transplant. But the sad fact was they could not get him in remission, so he was not eligible for a second transplant. There was no more treatment left for him.

"He's in room 11 with his partner Michael and his brother Steve," she said. "They are all shell-shocked at this news. It just makes me sick, Debra. They are such wonderful guys—they're architects. I thought maybe you could talk with them. I told them you were coming."

This was the "oh-shit-there's-no-hope-call-the-chaplain" situation. I don't get many calls like this because I usually know the patients. It's often much easier to discuss your impending death with someone you know. But this time I decided to make the fact I was a total stranger work for me.

When I walked in I said, "Hi, I'm Debra. I know I'm a total stranger, and you don't know me from Adam. But sometimes people find it helpful to sort things out with someone they *don't* know."

I intentionally used the phrase "sort things out" instead of "talk." "Talk" as in, "Don't you think you should 'talk' to someone?" always sounded patronizing to me. I liked the idea of having someone help me sort out my feelings, my questions, and my hopes—like cleaning out a drawer or organizing a closet.

I looked around the room and saw everyone had a bottle of water, and there was an extra one for me on the counter. There was also a big box of tissues next to my water bottle. Bottles of water and tissues are not good signs. It indicates you are going to cry—so much you'll need to rehydrate yourself.

Robert had no hair, but I could tell from his eyes and skin that his hair had been red. He wore gray flannel pants and a forest green shirt with woven stripes. Except for the fact that he was bald and a little thin, he looked fantastic.

So Robert, Michael, Steve, and I "sorted things out."

I turned to Steve. "Who's older, you or Robert?"

"I'm younger, younger than Michael, too. But they're both like brothers to me." Then he started to cry, and Michael reached over and squeezed his arm. I had a déjà vu feeling and realized this was the exact same room in which Lynie, Wes, and I sat talking with my oncologist.

Stay centered.

"I just want you all to know that I'm not afraid of dying," Robert said. It felt as if he was trying to stop the flow of tears, reassuring everyone.

"So what do you think happens when you die?" I asked.

"Steve and I weren't raised with any religion at all. But I came very close to death during my transplant. I know what it's like. There was a big wide doorway. I wanted to walk through, but I couldn't because it wasn't yet my time. But it was beautiful and peaceful. Really it was."

This made all of us cry, not because he seemed brave or courageous, but because he was so sincere and so badly wanted to comfort his family.

"You know how hard the transplant was," he continued. "It was horrible—the worst thing that I've ever gone through. Death will not be horrible. I just wish I didn't have to leave you."

They sat there and cried for a while, and I took deep breaths and calmed myself down. I knew part of my reaction was deep gratitude that my family and I had a very different conversation in this room. When it looked as if everyone was breathing again, I asked, "So Robert, what was your life like before all this?"

He told me he and Michael were moving to London because he was starting a job in an architectural firm there. They had met in college and had been together for ten years.

Michael jumped in. "We had our stuff packed. The movers were coming the next day. Robert had gone in for a blood test because he wasn't feeling well. His neck hurt. We never thought . . ."

Almost nobody thinks it's cancer. They think it's an infection, the flu, a cyst, a pulled muscle, or like me, they didn't have any symptoms. It's right to think it's something common, innocuous. If you thought every cough and ache was cancer, you'd go nuts. I think this is why there usually is such a shock.

In medicine they say, "Common things happen commonly," and "When you hear hoof beats, think horses, not zebras." This is to keep doctors from going immediately to a wild or exotic diagnosis. But there are times the test shows an uncommon thing has happened. Robert showed up with a zebra, not a horse.

In spite of all the tears, my sense of them was they were quite grounded, accepting, and not fighting the news. But I knew how hard it was to be in the No Clue Zone. There was a change of plans, but a change to what?

"Robert," I said, "I guess the question for you now is, what do you want the rest of your life to mean?"

"Yeah, you're not dead yet!" Steve quipped. We all starting laughing because we all knew the Monty Python line from *The Life of Brian*. The laughter came at just the right moment because we needed a break from the sorrow and the grief. And the crying—you have to stop at some point just because you get a headache, and you get really dehydrated. And Steve was right; Robert wasn't going to die immediately.

"That's what I can't believe," Robert said. "I feel so well right now. It's unbelievable that the cancer is back. I can hardly think about what I want the rest of my life to mean."

"This isn't something you have to answer right now," I said. "It's something to think about. And you may want to think about with whom you want to spend your remaining time. Terminal illness is an even better excuse than cancer for dropping relationships."

Robert nodded. "That's excellent news. I think I'll let my PBS pledge go." He stared out the window for a moment and then turned to Steve and said, "But how—what are we going to tell Mom and Dad? Mom will scream."

"His parents have been great," Michael said. "But they had so much hope. He's not kidding—his mother will start screaming. This will kill her. How are we going to tell her?"

"Mothers are notoriously hard to control," I said. "Especially their emotions. So you might think about getting into a mental/emotional place where you are very calm and grounded. Then decide that however she reacts is okay with you. It's been my experience the more relaxed you are, the calmer the other person can be." I was thinking about how I yawned while Charlotte was in hysterics.

"I do meditate," Robert said. "I know how to get myself in a centered space." He paused for moment. "But do you think it's wrong to hope for a miracle?"

"It's never wrong to hope for a miracle," I replied. "It's not an either/or situation. So on one hand you can accept the medical reality, and on the other you can hope for a miracle. Do both."

I cracked open my water bottle, and on cue we all took drinks.

"Like gazelles at the watering hole," I said and then held the tissue box out for everyone. It felt as if I were celebrating Communion: tissues and water instead of bread and wine. I did feel in communion with them. How could I not after being with them in the most vulnerable of places—talking about death?

We talked some more about Robert continuing to do the things that gave him joy and fed his soul. He had a huge network of friends and family, so I wasn't worried that they would be alone in this. I gave them each my card and a hug and encouraged them to call me anytime.

"I'll keep you in my prayers," I said.

I opened the door and was just about to walk out when Robert asked, "What can you tell me about actually dying?"

Argggh—the Doorknob Confession! This is anything that is said just as you have your hand on the doorknob to leave, which then makes it impossible to go. Examples of this include, "I killed my stepfather," "God told me to tell you something," "My sister takes my pain pills," and everyone's favorite, "I know what happened to Jimmy Hoffa."

I closed the door and sat back down. "Well, do you want to die at home?" I asked.

Robert nodded. I could see the question shocked them because I asked it as casually as, "Do you like Chinese food?"

"So if you want to die at home," I said, "it's a good idea to call hospice. Your case manager can give you the number and—"

"But what about the actual dying?"

"So you might go into a coma—"

"I mean the spiritual part."

"Oh. You have a better clue than I do. You had the near death experience."

"Yes, the doorway, it was really more of an archway—a Romanesque archway. Are you familiar with that?"

"Like the Bernard Maybeck First Church of Christ Scientist in Berkeley?"

"My God! You know it? Yes, exactly, that's Romanesque—although now that I think about it, the arch that I saw when I was near death was more like the Moissac Abbey at Tarn-et-Garonne in France."

I kicked myself. I knew nothing about architecture, but I couldn't resist showing off the only architectural fact residing in my brain, and now we were totally off track.

"How do you know the Maybeck church?" he asked.

"I went to UC Berkeley and walked by it nearly every day." I paused, thinking hard. "But I never knew the archway looked like the entrance to the afterlife." That ought to get us back on track.

Michael cleared his throat. "The Maybeck church is really considered to be eclectic Craftsman with Romanesque and Gothic motifs."

It was Steve who got us back on track. "I can't believe we're sitting here talking about *architecture* when Robert, when Robert is going to . . ."

"Die," I finished for him. Then everybody started crying again. We were out of water now. Robert stood up and said, "Perhaps I'm going to die from this at some point, but right now I'm starved. Let's go eat!" And like a congregation preparing to hear the benediction, we all stood.

We had another round of hugs and good-byes. Then we all went to lunch.

The conclusion of this visit may seem abrupt and unbelievable, and that is the operative word. The previous hour was so unreal to them that going for lunch was simply like going out after a movie. I knew our conversation felt like something they watched—like it never really happened at all.

Cheerful or Fearful?

My first clue that some people would have trouble with my attitude came to me before I was even diagnosed. I was talking to a fellow chaplain just after my biopsy. He seemed not to believe me when I said, "I've led a charmed life. Shit happens. There's no reason why I shouldn't have some shit in my life."

He did a double take and said something about me being
angry, but I really wasn't. I said, "Look, I've been a chaplain for
twenty years. I've contemplated my own death every day. I'm not
saying that I won't be upset if they tell me I have cancer, but I'm
not angry."

Then, after my diagnosis, a colleague from work called and
said, "Of course you're freaking out."

"Not really," I said. I thought she was projecting. I didn't say
that because in the same way that proclaiming you're not insane
makes everyone think you really *are* insane, strongly proclaiming
that you are okay makes everyone think you're in denial.

Robert did not fear dying because he felt that compared to his
experience of a transplant, death would be easy.

What many people didn't realize was that cancer was not the
worst thing that ever happened to me—getting fired many years
ago was worse. I know. You're shocked. How could losing a job be
worse than cancer?

The Theory of Relativity

I had been working for seven years as a spiritual counselor for a
Seattle hospice program. It was a job I loved. My colleagues and
I had a mutual love and respect for one another, and I looked
forward to going to work every day. I loved introducing myself
to people as a "hospice spiritual counselor." (Just say the word
"hospice" and you are immediately thought of as "special" because
people are so freaked out about death.)

All you need to know is that they fired me because of a book
I wrote and that I felt betrayed.

On the afternoon it happened, I was in such a state of shock,
I saw nothing odd about keeping my appointment with Nello, my
hairdresser.

I settled myself into Nello's chair and he fluffed up my hair the way hairdressers do. "So I bring you a glass of wine I know you love. But first, how are you, Debra?"

"Just got fired, Nello." I looked at my watch. "About twenty minutes ago." He looked horrified and his hands froze on my head so that my hair looked big and scary like a head full of snakes.

"I go get you wine." He brought me an enormous glass of chardonnay. I must have been reeking of need because he massaged my scalp and my neck and my shoulders and my arms and hands. Then he gave me the most precise haircut I've ever had. It felt as if he were cutting each hair individually. I was in that chair for two hours.

Little did I know that a voice mail about my termination had already been sent out to the hospice team, and they were calling my house and leaving messages like, "I just heard the news, and I can't believe they terminated you!"

"Debra, getting fired over a book is noble. Call me."

"I'm shocked. I'm so shocked. Call me."

Wes came home to all those messages and since it was after eight o'clock by that time, he wondered where I was. When I finally drove up in the driveway, he came running out.

"Where have you been?"

"Getting my hair cut."

"There are all these messages about you being fired, and I was worried you went to a bar."

"A bar? Oh, sweetheart, you know I'd go to a bakery before a bar any day."

In the days that followed I kept reliving the termination scene. I sobbed every day for hours. "It's all my doing. I've ruined my life!" I said to Wes. I was inconsolable.

Getting fired is nothing like getting laid off or having your company go under. There is something particularly shameful and humiliating about it. It also brought up the whole identity question: If I couldn't continue to do my job, then who was I? Do I have any worth if I can't do my job? For many months afterward when people asked what I did, I said, "I'm a hospice spiritual counselor." I clung to that job title like a life raft. But it was a raft with a slow leak, and I knew that I had to eventually let go of it.

I was not a spiritual counselor anymore, but I was still a writer! And then the unthinkable happened. My publisher pulled out. So I gave birth to a book into which I poured my heart and soul—and it was stillborn. This put me into a downward spiral of such raw grief and anguish that I thought it would kill me.

I was not a hospice spiritual counselor. I was not a writer. I was not.

Since I couldn't face being, I got into doing. I madly did projects around the house. I painted the deck and put in a new garden. I spray painted the lawn furniture. I brushed our dog daily until she was nearly bald. I volunteered at our local public television station. Physically I was healthy, but emotionally and spiritually I was ready for the ICU. Unless you are healthy in all three areas, you aren't really healthy.

When you lose your job, people don't continue to call and ask how you're doing. They don't send cards and flowers. They don't bring over food, although I was so paralyzed with grief that I couldn't even go out grocery shopping. I was sure the checker would take one look at me and know that I had lost my job.

It wasn't the kind of thing where I could stand up in church and say, "I'd like prayers for myself because I was terminated from my job." I couldn't even enter the sanctuary, but stood in the narthex weeping and shaking. I was ordained in this church and felt that I had let down the entire congregation. The few people who knew were loving and supportive, but I was too scared and ashamed to ask for prayer.

The day after I was fired, an acquaintance called and asked, "So have you got your résumé out there yet?"

That was like asking a widow the day after her husband's funeral if she had any dates lined up. The acquaintance didn't want to be with me in my pain, and he wanted to fix it. To him it was just a job. To me it was my identity and a huge part of my life.

Of course, I was furious with Mr. Martha Miyagi because I had felt called by the Spirit to write that book. And now look! I was mad as hell and confused. What was I supposed to do now? I didn't know that the real question was, who was I supposed to be?

After a while, I knew I had to process this whole experience so I started talking about it—incessantly. Whenever I met someone new, or someone who didn't yet know, I went into the whole story. Misunderstood and betrayed! Deceit and duplicity!

After a while, I noticed that Wes and others who had heard it would move away when I started my story. That is when I learned the difference between venting feelings and feeding feelings. There came a certain point when I realized that every time I told the story, I was actually nursing my anger, hurt, and resentment. So I just shut up.

I began taking a two-hour yoga class. When the teacher asked us to go around and say why we came to the class, I simply said, "I came here to heal."

I also started meditating every day. This was unbearably painful at first because I mentally flogged myself for having been so brainless about the book. My first mantra was something like, "Goddamn stupid idiot." After a while I stopped that and instead alternated between, "Lord Jesus Christ, have mercy on me," and the Buddhist, "Om Mani Padme Hum."

The Buddhist mantra literally means, "Hail! The jewel in the lotus." That just got me thinking about jewelry or how I should be out in my garden. So I chose to focus on the interpretation that said the mantra helps you achieve perfection in the practice of generosity, ethics, tolerance and patience, perseverance, concentration, and wisdom. And who couldn't use a little more of all that?

Eventually my mind settled down and I would get brief glimpses of peace; a hint of serenity here and there, an occasional faint feeling of self-acceptance.

I did not go through this experience with anything resembling grace and charm. I definitely lost my inner joy for a while. It was two years before I was able to introduce myself simply as "Debra Jarvis," without some feeble tagline about being a writer or a hospice spiritual counselor. It was four years before I knew I was valuable and loved just because I existed—just because I *was*.

I mention all this so you understand what I had under my belt before my cancer diagnosis.

My cancer diagnosis was not a moral or ethical dilemma. Cancer is a disease and disease happens. Nobody betrayed me. Family and friends were there for me—even if some of them thought I was in denial.

Bad Luck, Sorrow, and Grief

It is possible to be betrayed and get cancer at the same time. This is what happened to Rick.

I first met him during a fire drill at the clinic. When the drill begins, everyone on the floor has to leave the building and go stand outside in the parking lot. The only exception is if you are doing direct patient care. So the alarm went off. It was cold. It was rainy. I'm a weenie. I saw the floor monitor coming down the hall, and I ducked into a room. Sitting hunched over in the bed was a man about thirty. He had white blonde hair and light blue eyes.

"Hi, mind if I hide out in your room?"

He started laughing. "Sure, be my guest." I closed the curtains to his room. "So that makes me an accomplice," he whispered.

"Yes, it does," I whispered back. "I'm Debra, one of the chaplains."

"I'm Rick. If anyone comes to get you, you can pretend to be absolving me."

"Okay, but first I have to hear all your sins."

He looked at his watch and gave me a big grin.

He was adorable. And he was Catholic, I was sure of it. Protestants don't talk about their pastors absolving them—unless he was Episcopalian.

"I do accept indulgences," I said, intentionally using the Catholic term, "indulgences."

"I got some old lottery tickets. Will that get me out of purgatory?"

"Ah-ha! You *are* Catholic."

"Was."

"So where are you now with all that?"

"I would say that I'm spiritual, not religious. I believe that there is a Higher Power. I pray, and that's all I want to say."

"Spiritual not religious." I hear this every day. I think people say this for many different reasons. They've had a bad experience with their childhood church, but they still believe in God. Or they are agnostic and want to keep their options open. Or they want to get you off their backs. I knew if I talked with Rick long enough, all that would unfold.

I kept waiting for him to straighten up, but he stayed hunched over.

"Okay, so what brings you to our fine establishment? I know it's not the lunches." He laughed.

"Oh, just a little sarcoma here in my shoulder." It was then that I realized he *was* sitting up and that the hunch was an enormous tumor. He looked like he was wearing football pads on one shoulder. It took me a few moments to take it all in. "It's kinda big," he said apologetically.

"Are we giving you chemo?" I asked.

"I was getting chemo, but now I come in every day for a dressing change.

On cue his nurse came in. "Alrighty, are you ready?" I knew she said this for my benefit and to give him a moment to ask me to leave if he wanted.

"Do you mind if I stay?" I asked.

"If you can stand it. It's pretty disgusting," he said.

"Oh, I love gross, oozing wounds."

His nurse carefully peeled off the old dressing which was wet and yellow. I peered over her shoulder. He was right. It was disgusting—raw and bloody and oozing yellow pus. The wound was big, about the size of a pie plate. She had a hard time keeping the gauze on because his shoulder was so misshapen and it was too painful to stick anything to his skin. It was almost as if he needed something he could wear tight against him that could keep the dressing in place. Something like a tight and stretchy vest. Hey . . . I could make a tight and stretchy vest.

After work I drove straight to the fabric store. I flipped through the pattern books until I found a simple vest. It was so simple it was dorky, but it would be perfect for my purposes. Spandex—nix the sparkly kind, something manly, not too medical looking. I found a green/blue tie-dye piece of Spandex that was pretty low key. The blue matches his eyes, I thought. I knew he couldn't manage zippers and buttons, so I bought Velcro tape to close it.

When Wes came home that night I was sitting at my serger.

"You're sewing?" he asked.

"Special project. I'm almost done."

I finished it that night and took it in to work with me the next morning. I showed his nurse. "Oh, my gosh, it's perfect!" she said.

When Rick came in for his dressing change I was right there. I couldn't wait to show him. "Ta-da!" He blinked and looked confused. "I call it the Bandage Vest," I said putting it on. "Except it will be very snug on you and hold the dressing in place."

"Thanks. I—I don't know what to say."

"'Thanks' is good. So you weren't here long enough yesterday for me to hear your whole story. How were you diagnosed?"

I settled back in a chair with coffee in my red commuter cup.

"I'm not really from Seattle. I'm really from Virginia . . ." He kept talking, but I couldn't keep my eyes off his vest. It held the dressing in place and didn't hurt his skin like the adhesive. I'd made the armholes really big so that the tumor would fit through. The color was perfect for him. Maybe I should patent it?

". . . so first they told me I had cancer, then they told me I had AIDS."

"What?" Jerked out of my self-adoration, I choked on my coffee and started coughing.

"Yeah. But the cancer, the AIDS, that wasn't the worst part. The worst part was that my girlfriend Leslie didn't tell me she was HIV positive. She didn't know how much I loved her. She was afraid I would reject her, so she just walked out and never came back. But I loved her, and if she had gotten sick I would have taken care of her."

"Oh, my God, Rick! That is just a *bit* much. What's getting you through this, because you are totally off the stress scale."

"I don't know. I just keep going and praying."

I knew he didn't want to talk about his prayer life so I couldn't bring that up. What about his girlfriend? "Does Leslie know she infected you?" I asked.

"Yeah, I called her in Virginia and told her everything."

"What did she say?"

"She was crying on the phone, she was really upset and couldn't talk. I tried calling her back. For days I kept calling. Finally someone answered—her landlord."

"So she moved out?"

"No. She killed herself."

This last revelation stunned me into silence. We didn't speak for a long time. Rick just stared down at the blankets on the bed, and I looked out the window. I wondered what had happened to Leslie that she didn't realize this wonderful man loved her? Or was she so wounded that she felt she was unlovable? And who had wounded her?

Finally he spoke.

"It was the betrayal that hurt the most. Have you ever been betrayed?"

"Yes. It's excruciating."

"And you wonder if you can trust anyone ever again."

I had no wisdom, no advice, no useful information to give him. But I could witness his suffering, and that in itself was healing. In spite of my having been mentally absent for a few moments, I had never gone so deeply with a patient so quickly. I think it happened because on some subconscious level, both Rick and I knew he had so little time.

When I saw him the next week, he wasn't wearing the vest because it was now too small for him. His tumor was doubling every twenty-four hours. He could no longer move his arm, and he begged the doctors to cut it off.

The part of his story I missed was that both his parents were dead, and he was diagnosed when he was out here on vacation, so he just stayed in Seattle.

The last time I saw him was in the hospital after he'd had surgery to remove his arm, his shoulder and the bulk of the tumor that was growing through his rib cage. By that time he had metastases to his brain and couldn't talk. He died two days later.

For the next few weeks I chose to believe in Heaven because I wanted Rick to be together with Leslie. I wanted Heaven to be like a Versed/Fentanyl IV drip where you awaken and forget all your painful experiences on Earth. I wanted them to be healthy and in one another's arms, loving and forgiving.

And I wanted Jesus to be there with a big smile and say, "Welcome! What brings you to our fine establishment? I know it's not the lunches."

Bratitude

I knew that many people didn't know about these experiences I had with people who seemed to have all the bad luck, sorrow, and grief in the world. But many of them did know and still didn't understand why I wasn't furious or miserable about my own diagnosis.

Sometimes I felt as if they were trying to provoke me into anger or depression: "But you're in such good shape and so healthy and it *still* didn't prevent you from getting breast cancer."

It's true that I exercised and ate boatloads of salmon and broccoli, and drank green tea and kefir, and took vitamins and supplements, and went to church and yoga classes, and read the *New Yorker*. But I did all that because it felt good, not because I was trying to prevent cancer.

I don't think I'm being Pollyanna (talk about denial!) when I say I had lots for which to be grateful. I was the poster child for early detection through mammogram. I had an early stage cancer even though it got upgraded to Stage II. I had only *one* positive lymph node out of three. I didn't have a tumor that was doubling every twenty-four hours.

Not only had I seen people come in with much worse cancer than me, but what about people all over the world who don't even get diagnosed, let alone treated?

I'll admit that I sometimes get impatient when I hear patients complaining about their treatment. I've asked more than once, "Do you *not* want to be treated?" So far no one has slugged me, because I say it gently, and only after I'm sure they're done venting and are now on to actually feeding their frustration.

The other thing I get impatient about is doctor bitching. It's so easy to be angry with doctors when you can't think of anyone else to dump on. "Now my doctor won't give me chemo because my counts are low! Now my doctor is putting me on antibiotics because I've got an infection!" These are examples of things that are not within a doctor's control.

I hear stuff like this all the time, and when I do I ask, "Of course you know your doctor can't control that, so what are you really upset about?"

The answer is often, "Having cancer." So we go from there.

Medical errors, however, are a different deal, although most doctors do not set out to intentionally ruin your day. Be as pissed off as you want about screw-ups, but still remember that like the rest of us, physicians would like to be flawless.

I knew my surgeon did the best he could to get my port-a-catheter line into my subclavian. I had a funky vein, perhaps it zigged where it should have zagged—whatever. It was as if he encountered road construction and had to take a different route. I learned that not every medical procedure can go as planned.

Here is something else I learned from that experience: never wear fancy panties to the hospital—especially ones with bright red poppies on them. Because when I woke up in the recovery room and sat up to barf, the back of my gown opened up. The nurse looked at my panties and screamed, "She's bleeding!"

And my Wes, who is, uh, *familiar* with my underwear, said, "No, no, it's her panties. They're poppies!" He was quite pleased with himself that he could identify the flower.

It's Only Temporary

Just before I was diagnosed, I was given a beautiful temporary office. It was temporary because at some point a much bigger wig than I would be hired, and she or he would move in there. Actually, I wasn't even a wig—more of a hairpiece.

This office not only had a window, but a small round table with two chairs, a long expanse of desk space and a giant filing cabinet. Space was at a premium at the clinic. Think apartments in Manhattan. So it was unbelievable that the chaplain would get this fabulous space.

How did I get this office? The manager of that floor took pity on me because she heard how one day I was wandering through the clinic like Moses in the Sinai, looking for a place to have a confidential conversation with a terminally ill patient. But she warned me that I could be tossed out at any moment.

"Just like life," I said.

At first I just brought in my desk supplies and protein bars. I was afraid to really move in, because who knew when I would be asked to move out? Then one day, one of the infusion nurses stopped by and said, "Debra, you need to fully inhabit this office! It's all yours."

She was right. I knew I was going to die someday, but that didn't stop me from living. So what was I waiting for? I hung some art, and brought in a lamp, a table runner, my raku jar, and a teapot with Japanese teacups.

I made tea for everyone who came in for an appointment. We sat at the little round table and talked. People loved it because it didn't feel medical. It felt special. I loved every moment in that office and was so glad that I moved in.

Two months later I was diagnosed and then off six weeks recuperating from surgery. A few days before I was to return, I received a voice mail telling me that they had just hired someone who would be taking the office and that I needed to vacate.

Wes helped me move out, filling a box with my books and emptying the desk drawers. I was wrapping my raku jar in bubble wrap. This was a gift from my hospice team, and they had filled it with their written blessings. They gave it to me after I was fired.

Wes looked up from the box he was packing. "I'm so sorry, baby. I know you loved this office, and you really made it your own."

I placed my raku jar in the box and said, "You know, it's okay. It's not the worst thing that ever happened to me."

Five

CHEMO SAVVY

Dear Family and Friends,

I see most of you some of the time, but some of you none of the time. So I thought I'd send an update, especially because I've been getting worried calls from folks who thought perhaps I was rolling in vomit, which I'm not.

First of all, I have absolutely no regrets that I have chosen to receive my care at the Seattle Cancer Care Alliance. Not only is it ridiculously convenient (I walk to the desk and get my wristband), but I can also guiltlessly eat all the cookies I want on Thursday afternoons. Plus, I get to see many of my co-workers, and we laugh, joke, and they bring me more cookies and bottled water.

Yes, it was weird at first. But after the staff and I all agreed that it *had* to be weird, it was much easier. Susan G., R.N., who after vowing total love and commitment, and promising to be gentle and take it out if I didn't like it, was the one who accessed my port for the first time. Like many women, I closed my eyes, and it was over before I knew it.

Before my actual chemo infusion, there was a tearful moment between my nurse Sherry and me. It brought up those questions: How could this happen to one of our own? How do we care for one of our own? Of course, it does happen, and has happened, and I'm afraid to say, statistically will happen again. But I'm happy to say that not only *can* we care for our own, but we also do it very well. I never had any doubts.

Regarding the Area Formerly Known as My Breast: Last week I assembled a crack team of objective female nurses. Using modern scientific theories and methods including the Krebs cycle, quantum mechanics, Avogadro's hypothesis, the laws of thermodynamics, and string theory, the consensus was: "Close enough."

So in a couple of weeks, I will be getting that hateful implant port removed. It sticks out of the side of my "breast" like a nasty cigarette butt, and I can't wait to be rid of it. Now I know that no doctor, nurse, or chaplain gets up in the morning and says, "Hmm, how can I wreck someone's day? Can I possibly inflict more pain than necessary?" Nevertheless, I am madly hoping that this procedure goes smoothly.

Chemo comments: My daily oral Cytoxan tablets are a beautiful robin's egg blue. I call them, "Pills of Light and Consciousness." My daily Protonix, which stops acid production in my stomach, are the "Pills of Compassion." So I leave the house in the morning feeling quite enlightened. I am a little more tired these days, but I truly think it's vicarious fatigue from watching the Tour de France. I find the Alps particularly exhausting.

We have hit upon the right medication for my nausea, which of course, is the most expensive medication. I call these the "reindeer pills" because their name sounds like something Santa Claus would shout from his sleigh: "Ondansetron!" (aka Zofran). Also they keep anything from flying up out of my stomach. I take these for the three days after my infusion, and I'm just fine. I am truly grateful to the pharmaceutical wizard who came up with these babies.

I am also truly grateful to co-workers, friends, and family who bring meals, grocery shop, provide amusing toys (what would I do without Space Mucous?), and weed our garden. This afternoon, I received a totally unsolicited bowl of fresh marinara sauce, pasta, and a berry pie! And I so appreciate the hilarious cards, phone calls, dog portraits, and drawings.

Last week our water heater blew up. I went down into the basement, and floating toward me in four inches of water, was my SCCA portable picnic blanket. (It floats!)

It was 6:30 in the morning, Wes had already left for work, and I couldn't lift the boxes around the water heater to shut it off. My neighbor arrived in record time, turned it off, and then vacuumed out all the water. Wes, having just arrived at work, turned right around, and furiously pedaled home again.

Other neighbors came over immediately to help me separate *hundreds* of dripping photographs, and lay them out to dry. The photos covered our entire living room floor. It was an involuntary life review as I was forced to look at high school high jinks, old boyfriends, and regrettable pictures from UC Berkeley.

As painful as this was, I was able to detect the presence of some Unseen Hand in even the most distressing periods of my life. It's a Presence that I feel now, made known not only through the people in my life, but also through easy-to-miss signs and miracles.

The latest was on the Fourth of July. Wes and I have regularly been doing a two hundred-step stair-climb down to the Burke-Gilman Trail. It is lush with ferns and ivy and overhung with cedar and fir boughs.

On the cool early morning of the fourth, we noticed that someone (A mad artist? A cranky child?) had spilled green glitter down the stairs. It was beautiful—as if some mystical pixie had come and blessed us. People going up and down had tracked the glitter all the way to the bottom. Panting and puffing on my way up I remarked to Wes, "It's hard to see the glitter on every step. But it's there if I look carefully."

And that is how I feel about this cancer experience: It's hard to see the glitter on every step. But it's there if I look carefully.

Love and Hugs,
Debra

The Angle on Angels

I was sitting out in the infusion floor waiting room with Ellen. She had been coming in for years to get infusions. The waiting room looks out on Lake Union and beyond that you can see Queen Anne Hill and beyond that, because it was a gorgeous, blue sky day, you could see the Olympic mountains. I think it is so cool that they gave the best view to the patients and not the administrators. I asked Ellen to tell me what happened when she received her diagnosis.

"It was in the morning," she said. "I made my doctor promise, no matter what the results were, that he would call. So the phone rang and it was him and he told me I had breast cancer and that it was advanced. After I hung up I closed my eyes for a minute—I was trying to take everything in. When I opened them again, the sun was streaming through the French doors onto the hardwood floors. The light was very bright, unusually bright, and the wood looked golden. I stood up, and that was when I felt them around me—angels.

"I walked down the hall to my bedroom, I could feel them following me—there was more than one. It was almost as if I could hear them, but no, it was a sense I had of their presence. I felt very calm and at peace. I knew whatever happened I would be okay."

In the Bible, angels usually have three different jobs: guardians, as in the angels with Daniel in the lion's den; messengers, like Gabriel who gave Mary the results of her pregnancy test, and terminators, like the angels who arrived to destroy Sodom and Gomorrah. Perhaps this variety keeps them from getting bored and looking for a different life altogether, in, say, the travel industry.

Like Ellen's, the angel stories I hear are mostly of the guardian/ messenger category. I'd like to think they've moved out of the terminator business, but I can't be sure. So I asked some doctors about angel stories, and they told me they rarely hear them, or if they do, they don't get the gory details.

A cardiologist told me that he had a patient who had a heart valve replacement who he expected to sail through the surgery. But day after day he continued to go downhill.

"Then one day, I walk in, and the guy is sitting up in bed. I ask, what happened? He told me matter-of-factly that he had a vision the night before who told him he could choose to get well or die— his choice. So he chose to get well. But he didn't say who it was."

I bet the guy had an angel drop by, but he wasn't comfortable telling his doctor, a "man of science." But patients figure this is my department, so I hear about angels all the time. A patient's daughter told me she was so stressed out by her mother's cancer that she thought she was just going to break down, have a heart attack, and die.

"I was sitting in the surgery waiting room with my head down, my eyes clenched shut, and my hands in fists on my lap. Then I felt these warm soft wings surround me from behind. It was the most wonderful feeling. I don't know how long it lasted, but gradually I realized that I was looking at my hands resting open in my lap. The feeling stayed with me for the longest time. Now anytime I started to tense up, I remember the feeling of those wings around me."

I have never seen an angel myself, but I think sometimes, it's just that I don't recognize them. Or they are invisible. I have had that experience. One day, B.D. (before diagnosis), I was out running and came to an intersection. I don't know if I was zoned out or what, but I started to run through the intersection without even looking. And then it was as if a giant arm reached out and stopped me. I came to a sudden stop just in time to have a car roar by, inches away from me. Every time I walk through that intersection I am reminded of that.

I had a patient who would say to me, "Debra, everyone who walks in the door has a message for me from God. You must be alert! Angels are everywhere. You must look for the divine, search for it, insist on finding it!"

And a little while later I was grocery shopping, and the guy asked, "Paper or plastic?" And I thought, "Paper or plastic?" There was that sturdy brown paper bag looking so grounded and sensible. Was that the message? Then there was the floaty white plastic bag, so ephemeral, ethereal, almost intangible. Paper? Or plastic? In the end I had him put the paper in the plastic, thinking that perhaps the message for me was that I needed to integrate my life.

For years nurses have been called "angels of mercy." But I know this pisses off some nurses who are proud of their degrees and their technical skills. I think all this anger stems from misunderstanding angels.

First of all, by definition angels are more powerful and intelligent than humans. Second of all, the Biblical angels were not beings with whom you'd want to clash. They don't take any shit. Take a look at the story of Jacob who wrestled with an angel all night and was left with a permanent limp. I don't see many examples of angels being all that nice. Maybe when they were talking to the shepherds, "Fear not, I bring you glad tidings of great joy." I'd like to think they said that in a friendly, soothing tone, but who knows?

So I can see how easy it is to describe nurses as angels of mercy. Sometimes it felt to me as if the nurses were more powerful and intelligent than humans. And most of them certainly did not take any shit—not that any of them left their patients with a permanent limp or anything. And as for the "mercy" part, if you've ever had a nurse give you pain meds, you know how merciful it feels.

The problem lies in how angels are portrayed in figurines and Christmas cards, which make them look sweet, adorable, and lobotomized. Just remember that in the Bible, when people run into angels, they are usually awestruck.

Caring for Our Own

A few weeks after I was diagnosed, one of our infusion "angels of mercy" was also diagnosed with breast cancer. Unbelievable! It felt to many as if the fifth floor was under siege. Who would be next?

We weren't the first employees in the clinic to have cancer and chemotherapy, but we were the first from the infusion department. That's like the cardiologist having a heart attack, the surgical nurse needing surgery, or the psychiatrist having a breakdown. You get the picture.

Like me, the infusion nurse continued to work and received her chemo in the clinic. But unlike me, she was very private about it. She didn't tell her patients. She didn't send out updates. Everyone does it his or her own way, and I knew it would take more energy for me to keep my chemo secret, than to be open about it.

The first time I registered and received my wristband I certainly didn't feel like a patient. I felt more like I was playing the part of a patient.

When I went to my dentist—now *that's* when I felt like a patient. I was only slightly familiar with the dentist's office, the receptionist, the dental assistant, and for that matter, my dentist. There was a certain professional distance in my relationships with the staff there.

But at the clinic there was no distance. We were close. The nurses knew me first as a friend and colleague. I had shared meals, gone out for drinks, and attended parties with them. How can you "unknow" someone? They had seen and approved my bionic breast. There was no going backward from *that*.

Because I continued to work in the clinic, the nurses couldn't suddenly put a distance between us because we relied on one another for patient care.

But sometimes an emotional connection with another can complicate medical care. Chemo nurses often see patients every week, and it's easy for them to become close to their patients. It can get to a point where they care so much about a patient that it becomes very difficult to inflict pain like starting an IV.

They don't notice it at first because the connection doesn't happen right away. It's like the old story of putting the frog in a pot of cold water and then turning up the heat. He doesn't notice it right away and by the time he does, it's too late. I don't know who in the *hell* is making frog soup like this, but if I ever find out I'm calling the authorities.

Anyway, the nurses have told me that the anxiety and fear of causing pain can inhibit them from doing a procedure correctly. This has not prevented them from becoming close to their patients. If they are sure they will not be able to start an IV they will ask another nurse to do it.

The clinic administrators understood all this and were worried that it would be too stressful for the nurses to give chemo to their co-workers. They knew that the frogs were already in hot water. So there was a plan in place to have nurses from outside the clinic come in and give us chemo if our staff was unable to do it.

I didn't think about this at all, so at my first chemo I was like, "La-la-la-la-la! Bring on the cookies! Bring on the tea!" I sobered up when Sherry came in to start my infusion. Her eyes welled up and she said, "I just don't want to hurt you."

"Don't worry—I used the lidocaine cream. I won't feel a thing!" I thought she meant having to stick the needle in my port site. But then I realized that she was thinking about the chemo. We hugged each other, and I could feel in her body that she really wanted to cry. So we just held on to one another for a few moments. This was going to be harder than I thought.

The first few times were the hardest. The nurses looked stricken when they saw me coming down the hall wearing my patient wristband. "Take that off," one of them said. "I can't look at it." She was joking, but she was not joking.

Oddly, I almost always kept my staff badge on, and when pondering this I realized I was doing two things: (1) I wanted everyone to realize, that yes, even the staff at a cancer center can get cancer, and (2) I was not really a "patient."

It was like saying, "See? I'm wearing my ID badge so I'm still one of you." I felt that I could somehow comfort them by reminding them I was still me, doing my job, just stopped in for a little chemotherapy.

There begins the slippery slope of caring for your care providers. I knew all about how patients love to please their doctors. I've heard patients describe the most horrendous pain, constipation, or nausea, and when their nurses asked, "Did you tell your doctor about this?" The patients would say, "Well, no. I didn't want to mention it."

At times like that I wanted to shake these patients and ask, "Are you nuts? You've got to tell them—you're preventing them from giving you good care. This is what these guys are paid for!"

How could people be so crazy? Easy. I found myself doing it the first month of chemo. Even though she knew me first as a colleague and a friend, Sherry's job was to get "nursey" with me and in fact, every week she would say, "Now I have to ask all the nosey, nurse questions." Then she would ask about my bowels and my nausea, and did I have any mouth sores, and how was I sleeping, and did I have any pain?

"Great, great, everything is great." I answered her as if we had just met up at a party and she had asked, "How's it going?"

Thank God Wes was there—he was my guardian angel. He just looked at me and said, "She's had quite a bit of nausea and does have some sore areas in her mouth."

Oh, yeah—the nausea, the sores. I'm surprised he didn't say something about my sudden amnesia. This is another reason it's good to have someone with you who really knows what's going on—they keep you honest.

I soft-peddled my symptoms because I didn't want to sound like a whiner or a baby. I didn't want to cause anyone any trouble. I didn't want to make more work for Sherry. These reasons are ridiculous and showed that I was missing the whole point of health care. It's like going into a restaurant hungry and then not ordering any food because you don't want to bother the waiter or the chef. *Please.*

But here's the other reason I didn't speak up: I was a *caregiver* damn it, not a care receiver. Of course that was all in my mind, and my mind had become one of those cigar-smoking mobsters in a 1940s motion picture.

"*I'm* the giver here, see? Nobody gives to me, see? My boys might make trouble for you, see?"

Picture this: my heart rolling its eyes at my mind.

I knew that I had to allow myself to receive care to heal. It goes back again to the foot-washing scene with Jesus saying to Peter in essence, "Get over your pride and self-sufficiency."

It's easy for Christians to go overboard on, "It's more blessed to give than to receive." It can start to get competitive, who can give most? Adding up your good deeds becomes a point of pride. God forbid you would actually have to accept help!

That's why I love the stories about Jesus eating dinner at everyone's house, letting perfume be poured on his head, sending out the disciples for fish and loaves. I mean, you never see *him* cooking the meals or actually pulling in a net of fish, do you? The guy knew how to let other people love him!

I believe that when you refuse help when you need it, you are stunting the spiritual growth of another. That person doesn't get to feel the joy in giving. You don't get to feel your own humanity and gratitude by accepting. Here's the new motto: "It's blessed to give *and* receive."

So I was determined to receive care gratefully and to become adept at shifting from co-worker to patient, although I knew the nurses would never truly think of me as a patient. And that was all right with me.

An Angel by Any Other Name

I know from experience that as a chaplain, I didn't connect with everyone. Jackson was a good example, a sweet young guy with prostate cancer. By young I mean forty, which is a young (and bad) age at which to get prostate cancer.

The first time I met him he told me about working on a fishing boat in Alaska. I asked if there were many African Americans working up there and he said, no, he was the only one on the crew. "I don't understand why," he said. "Because you can make a lot of money."

He always came in with his mom, and she and I connected, but I felt bad about chatting with her as Jackson just stared at the wall. So I visited a few times and that was it. I had been on chemo for about a month and felt as if I was adjusting to it. I ate saltines and Lorna Doones all day long to keep my nausea down. One afternoon, miracle of miracles, I was all caught up on my charting and had nothing to do. I looked again at the schedule and saw that Jackson was coming in. "What the heck," I thought, "I'll give it another try."

It was pretty much the same story, he was blank and bored until I said something about being a writer. He sat up. "Did you say you're a writer? I'm a writer, too!"

What? How had I missed this? He told me how he went to the University of Washington and took a creative writing class with Charles Johnson and had written this story for which he received an "A" and wanted to turn it into a book.

"Wow," I said. "Bring it in! I'd love to see it." I hadn't forgotten my experience with Mr. Christos and inwardly vowed that I would say only positive things. The next week he brought in thirty pages. I had never seen him so animated or excited.

"I got my nephew's old computer and printer. Took me a long time to find the story, but I worked on it some more." He handed it to me proudly.

"I can't wait to read it," I said.

"You're gonna make some corrections, right? Help me improve it? Give me comments?"

"Uh—sure. Just little corrections."

So I took it home. He wrote a story about a young boy named Richard. Going by the fact that Richard was learning his times tables, he was in second or third grade. But his internal dialogue sounded like a philosophy professor on mushrooms. Richard and some of his schoolmates get asked to cut down a Christmas tree. Mike, one of the boys in the group, is Richard's archenemy.

The teacher gives them all axes. In my comments I said nothing about the wisdom and improbability of handing out axes to eight-year-olds. They go out into the woods and tension mounts. They find a rabbit, chase it, and Richard kills it by throwing his ax at it. Again, I made no comments on the likelihood of an eight-year-old being able to do this.

They make a fire, roast the rabbit, and eat it. They get thirsty from eating the rabbit. They go to steal some water from the garden hose of a white man who comes out with a shotgun and threatened to shoot them. Richard and Mike fight, Mike almost drowns, but another guy pulls him out of the river. They reminisce about their encounters with white people. These passages were violent and hate-filled, and I wanted to weep. It was painful to read.

The next week I gave the corrected copy back to him and his first question was, "How much in royalties do you think I'll make?" I explained to him that perhaps he was getting a little ahead of himself and that at this point, asking about royalties was like looking at a foal and asking where we should build the shelves for his Triple Crown trophies.

So every week I gave him back a corrected copy, and he would bring me his latest work plus the rewritten earlier stuff.

One week I said to him, "Jackson, it almost seems like you plugged every other word into your thesaurus and used the biggest one."

"I did!" he said proudly. "I just want to shine it up."

"Well, sometimes the simplest words are the best," I said carefully.

"Nah!"

I didn't argue with him because it wasn't important. What was important was the fact that he found a new meaning in his life, was getting up in the morning, was writing thirty pages per week, and was writing about things that were heavy on his heart: poverty, racism, rage, violence, and death.

His mother said to me, "He gets up every morning and *gets dressed* before he starts writing. He wasn't even getting dressed before."

Jackson had talked glowingly about Charles Johnson being his professor. That gave me an idea. "Jackson," I said, "I am acquainted with Charles Johnson. If I happen to run into him, may I tell him about your book and how I met you, here at the cancer center? Maybe give him your phone number?"

"Oh, yeah, sure!"

Of course I'd rather surprise him, but I couldn't tell Charles Johnson anything without Jackson's permission or I would go straight to HIPAA hell.

Here's how well I knew Charles Johnson: I had been in a stationery store one day and he was one aisle over from me talking to someone about which school he was sending his daughter to. Yeah, we were really close buds.

So I e-mailed him, explained the situation and would he consider calling Jackson?

He wrote back that he would love to. So this is where I think angels take on all kinds of different forms. Charles not only called Jackson, but he arranged for them to meet in his office. He sent Jackson a huge packet of writing exercises and essays, all things that he would give his graduate students.

Jackson came into the clinic the next week and said, "Professor Johnson called me." And then he sat there for my entire visit with this blinding grin on his face.

I think Charles, or Chuck as I started calling him after a few e-mail messages, was both a messenger and a guardian angel for Jackson. His message was, you are valuable, your writing is important. And as guardian he was like the angel in the lion's den because Jackson felt he had this important writer in his corner, and so his life was worth fighting for.

I don't know what this novel meant for Jackson. Only he could say what it meant for him, but here is what I wondered about: Jackson was one of the sweetest, most compliant and gentle men I had ever met. Was Richard, the brave, take-no-shit protagonist his alter ego? Was Mike, the archenemy, someone he really knew, or was it possible that Mike was the symbol of his cancer? So he was always fighting Mike and nearly destroying him.

The other thing I wondered about but am now sure of is that I was the only white person to hear his feelings about prejudice and racism. Every week he said to me, "I'm writing it like it really is!" And every week I grieved for the way he saw it.

I Walk Therefore I Am

I was more religious about my morning walk than I was about going to church. In July in Seattle it's light by 5:30 a.m. I loved getting out the door by 6:00 a.m. and walking what Wes and I referred to as the "Deer Loop." We called it that because atop one of the houses is a very realistic life-size deer. It's not clear why the deer is there 365 days a year, but we like it. Whenever we pass it, I wave and call out, "Hi, deer!" I love that it sounds as if I'm greeting a loved one.

I walk fast—fifteen-minute miles. Wes calls this Chihuahua walking because I'm short and take a lot of fast little strides.

I found these walks both grounding and energizing. Watching the changes in everyone's garden, hearing the flickers and the crows, reminded me that life continued on around me. There was more to the world than just my chemo, my job, and me. And then something else began to happen.

It all started with the new cedar fence.

At this point I had walked the Deer Loop over fifty times and was pretty familiar with everyone's yard. Since every day felt so unpredictable to me, I liked the predictability of doing the same walk every morning. So I would do the usual walk past the deer, half a mile later have my ten-minute love fest with Max the dog (whose owner refused to part with him), and then continue on.

The cedar fence appeared about three-quarters of the way through the walk. It had magically gone up in the twenty-four hours since I last walked by, and I smelled it before I saw it. When I came upon it I stopped dead in my tracks and took a deep breath. The fence was strong and handsome. Unlike, say, a white picket fence, which is prissy and demanding and hard to please.

The fence was made of carefully milled, cut, and nailed planks. It was just a cedar fence. But as I stood before it I could feel the power of the tree in the fence.

Look deeper and see out of what I am made.

It was Mr. Martha Miyagi and yet it was not exactly the same voice. It was the fence, no; it was definitely the Divine, the Presence, the Spirit. I didn't have time to stand there and contemplate this mystery because I had to get to work. So I hurried off.

Here in the Pacific Northwest, cedar is a big deal, especially to the Native Americans. They make totem poles, drums, baskets, clothes, and masks out of cedar. There is a story that the spirit of a powerful and loving medicine man resides in the cedar tree. I love this because we have several cedars in our yard, and I've always felt their power. Anyway, when cedar burns, the blaze reminds everyone of the tree's great healing power. The aroma of cedar reminds everyone of the medicine man's great love for his people. So that's why cedar is used to pray for people.

Later that day I met George, an elderly man with esophageal cancer. He was frail and bent over. He was pretty quiet with everyone, but since he was a new patient, I stopped by to say hi and introduce myself.

At first he didn't say much, but the television was on with a story about Iraq. This is how we got on the subject of war, and then he began telling me about being in World War II. He talked about seeing men die before his eyes, about staying in a foxhole for days, about not wanting to die.

As he talked, I saw that deep inside he was not weak and sick but strong and powerful. I could feel all the love in and around him. I saw the tree in the fence.

Look deeper and see out of what I am made.

"I'm not afraid to die now," he said. "But I hope this chemo works. There's still some livin' I want to do."

His hope for healing was not born out of fear of death, but love of life. This is a very good thing. When people love life more than they fear death, they come to treatment with open hands, open hearts, open eyes. When people fear death more than they love life, they come clinging and clutching and grasping. Holding the breath. Furrowing the brow.

"I've seen many people die, includin' my wife," he said. "And her spirit just sort of eased on out."

Before I left I squeezed his hand and said, "You are your own medicine man."

He nodded and gave me a big grin.

The cedar fence was the beginning of the Spirit speaking to me in ways other than the Mr. Martha Miyagi voice in my head. That still came through, too, but now I perceived the Divine in all kinds of different things.

What's in a Name?

Words are powerful. That's why people paste up affirmations on their bathroom mirrors like, "I accept myself just as I am." That's why people memorize scripture and poetry and mantras.

God said, "Let there be Light." And there was light.

"Lather. Rinse. Repeat." I never questioned it.

Words can call something into being. Words can also destroy.

"Hi, I'm here for my *poison*." I had a patient who used to say that every time he came in for his chemo. Then he'd paste a big bitter smile on his face. He was angry and depressed and his docs were having a hard time getting his side effects under control.

One day his daughter and two-year-old granddaughter came in with him. There was a lot of jostling around and rearranging of chairs, so he didn't make his usual dramatic announcement about getting his poison.

His granddaughter looked like she belonged in a Ralph Lauren ad. She had a nest of shiny dark curls surrounding her face, red cherubic lips, and stunning dark blue eyes. She was a gorgeous child, which made me immediately suspect she was a brat.

"Papa up," she said reaching her little arms toward him. I saw how he just melted when he lifted her up on the bed. She cuddled up next to him with her bottle and her blanket and he put his arm around her. His nurse started his chemo and left.

"Papa good juice," she said pointing to his IV line. Well, it's true that Doxil is red and really does look like juice.

He looked at her and laughed. "Yes, that's Papa's juice. Papa's good juice."

I changed my mind; she was not a brat but a heavenly angel. "Lo, I bring you glad tidings of good juice!"

After that day, I never again heard him call his chemo "poison." And you can say what you want about how they finally found the right anti-nausea drugs for him or adjusted his chemo, but he never again complained of nausea.

Then there's Linda who asks me to come in and bless her bags of chemo before hooking up. The nurse hands her the bag, she kisses it, she holds it out to me, and I pray over it. Then she whispers to it, "Do your stuff!" and hands the chemo back to her nurse.

I thought of my chemo as powerful memory juice that helped my body remember how to heal itself. They've shown that everybody gets abnormal cell growth every day and the body takes care of it. Maybe sometimes the body just forgets. So I went to sleep on chemo nights hearing my cells saying, "Oh, yeah—now I remember. Mm-hmm, that's right. Of course! It's all coming back to me. Oh, right!"

One night I went to sleep and heard a cell saying, "Dude— like, now I remember!" Must have been all those weekends on the beach in Santa Cruz.

The Housecreeper

It was true that after my port placement Wes was doing everything around the house. He said to me, "We should get a housekeeper."

I hated the idea of a stranger coming in my house and touching my stuff. It bugged the hell out of me! I wanted to clean my own house. But I couldn't.

There was something else too.

My maternal grandparents came to the United States from Spain via Hawaii. My grandfather worked in the pineapple and sugar cane fields. It was brutally hard work. When they moved to California, he worked as a school janitor and my grandmother worked in the cannery. They were hardworking people. Are you noticing how many times I use the word "work"?

I was around eight years old when Nana said a lady at the cannery knew someone who knew someone who had a *housekeeper*. "Can you imagine?" Nana said, her voice dripping with disgust, "She can't even clean her own house."

I gasped because Nana was so outraged, and all the other adults were shaking their heads and tsk, tsk, tsking. But I had watched the television show *Hazel* and thought it would be kind of fun to have a housekeeper. But now I could see how *wrong* that was.

To me getting a housekeeper was an admission of how lazy I was, how I didn't value my own house, how I thought I was too good for menial work, how I was a completely immoral and undisciplined person.

When I explained all this, Wes just closed his eyes and pinched the bridge of his nose.

I finally cracked when a friend pointed out how exhausted Wes looked. "Do it for him," she said. So I agreed.

We arranged to have the same housekeeper as my neighbor up the street. The housekeeper arrived at 6:30 a.m. with a friend, carrying buckets of cleaning products and her own vacuum cleaner. I was in the downstairs bathroom getting ready for work. But I could hear them talking and oh, my God—they were speaking Spanish. Well, why wouldn't they? They were from Guatemala.

But I knew my dead grandmother sent them to torment me. I felt sicker to my stomach than usual and slunk out of the house.

I had my chemo that afternoon, and it was after my infusion that we came home to the Spotless Sparkle Palace.

"Hey! This is great!" Wes said running his finger over a table. "They even cleaned the light bulbs and the lamp shades. Wow."

"Hmph," I said.

I looked at a plant that I usually kept on the side of the coffee table. It was now sitting smack in the middle of it. "Why is this *here*?" I asked sharply.

"This bathroom is so clean I could eat in here!" Wes crowed. You must understand that this was coming from an infectious disease doctor.

"I'm starting dinner," I announced. "Just a little pasta with sauce." I opened the oven. This morning it looked like a field of turds, covered with big brown lumps of burned on cake batter. Now it was gleaming. Where were the pans that I stored in there?

I put on a pot of water to boil and took out the spaghetti. A neighbor had brought over this unbelievable marinara sauce, and I couldn't wait to eat it.

I opened the refrigerator, and I felt as if I walked into the wrong classroom. Yes, it was clean, but why was the mustard jar on the door? And—what's this? The soymilk was cozied up against the barbecue sauce. Where was the marinara? I yanked open the crisper drawer which was now where the meat drawer should be. The marinara sauce was in there snuggling with two containers of cottage cheese. I should have known.

Where was the Parmesan? I frantically searched the shelves. Hot smoked paprika next to Mom's raspberry jam. Beer bottles randomly scattered around like hand grenades. Where's the Parmesan?

Don't forget to breathe. In-breath or out-breath?

Fennel and feta in the meat drawer. Salad dressing chatting up the yogurt! Soy sauce cavorting with the string cheese! "Where's the Parmesan?" I said aloud, my voice catching.

Wes came bounding up the stairs from the bedroom, "What, honey? Did you say something to me?"

I was standing paralyzed in front of the open refrigerator, and then I started crying. "Where's the Parmesan?" I wailed.

"It's right here." He reached over my head and grabbed the hunk of cheese from the top shelf.

"That's where the pickles go," I sniffled. He just wrapped his arms around me, and I cried all over his shirt. "Everything's rearranged," I whimpered. "My body is rearranged. My schedule is rearranged. My whole life is rearranged. And now our fridge is rearranged. I can't find anything in there. I'm lost." I cried while Wes cooked the spaghetti and heated the sauce and set the table and made the salad.

Then I just sat there feeling all crappy and whiny. It was about wanting things to be the way they used to be. It was about resisting what *is*, and being in the aforementioned mode of clinging, grasping, and clutching. I wasn't lost, just not going anywhere.

"Honey, what would you like to drink?"

"Water," I answered.

Then I got up, gave him a hug from behind, and poked my fingers under his shoulder blades looking for wings.

Six

TRIED IN VEIN

Dear Fabulous Family and Friends,

Is it possible that I cursed myself by saying in my last update that I hoped my next procedure went smoothly?

At 6:40 a.m. on July 21, I went into the UW Medical Center to have my breast implant port removed. This is the little thingy sticking out of the side of my "breast" through which my plastic surgeon filled my implant. This is not to be confused with my port-a-catheter, which is in my chest and is used for infusions thus saving me from the odious IV needle in the arm or hand.

The anesthesia resident came in to start my IV. "I have a port-a-cath!" I crowed. He shook his head and said he wanted to put it in my hand. "Okay," I sighed. Well, he must have thought I said, "Poke around several times in the back of hand, make a big hematoma, and cause me to scream.

The scream was involuntary—honest. Wes said I sounded just like our late dog Cokey (may she rest in peace) when he tried to cut her toenails. The resident started to come at me again and I shrieked, "I have a port! Use the port!"

Turns out he didn't know how to access my port, nor did my nurse. I guess they both missed that class. They found a nurse who sort of knew how, but she didn't have the right needle. She ended up using a 1.5-inch needle, which was w-a-a-a-y long. But in the end, I got that hideous breast port out, and I'm thrilled.

They left my port-a-catheter accessed, and when I arrived for chemo that afternoon I looked as if I had an oil derrick sticking up out of my chest. My nurses were duly horrified.

However, before I went to chemo, in my grogged-out state, I called my parents to say hi. They were not home so I left a message. On the message, I said it was Friday (it was Thursday) and I sounded as if I'd been run over several times by a garbage truck—or so I'm told. Because you see, after the traditional IV cocktail of two fingers Fentanyl, a splash of Versed, and a twist of lemon, I remember nothing.

The next morning my mother called and left a message in what my sister and I call her "panic voice."

"Debbie Lynn?" she said. "This is Mom. Call me."

I heard this and said to Wes. "Oh, my God. Something's happened. Somebody died. I'd better call her right now."

Mom: "Hello?"

Me: "Hi, Mom, it's me. How *are* you?"

Mom: "I'm fine, but how are *you*?"

Me: "I'm fine, but really, Mom, how are *you*?"

Mom: (starting to get annoyed) "I'm fine! We got your message."

Me: "What message?"

And that's the beauty of anesthesia.

So I'm done with procedures for a while, and it's going well, except for the teeny-tiny meltdown I had a few weeks ago. It was mainly tears and an inability to walk down the hall into my room for chemo. I believe my exact words were, "I don't want to do this anymore!"

I was feeling quite tragic, but I'm afraid I just sounded squeaky and whiny. (Good hamster names!) It was brought on mostly by lack of sleep and learning about the staff support group called, "Caring for Our Own."

The support is, as Martha Stewart says, "a good thing," and I'm proud to work in a place that cares so much about their employees. But knowing that I was one of "Our Own" caused me all kinds of irrational guilt. (It was so easy to make it all about me!) I know that this is crazy. It is like apologizing for causing my mother's labor pains. But perhaps that's why they invented Mother's Day. Or is it Labor Day?

Global Warming Department: What is the mystery behind this? I know exactly what's causing global warming: the female baby boomers are all in menopause. There are enough hot flashes around to melt the polar ice caps, boil the Arctic Ocean, and then make tea. Two weeks ago I awoke and wondered why the smoke alarm had not gone off, because surely the house was on fire. Silly me. It was just as my oncologist had promised: abrupt menopause.

The worst is not the hot flash, but the insomnia that follows. I'm so awake and alert I could hear a dog fart in Afghanistan. So in addition to the usual sleeping meds (mallet on the head, shot of tequila) I do what I often suggest patients do when they can't sleep: I pray. So just know that at some point, everyone getting this update has been prayed for.

My prayer is short, from the Buddhist tradition, and covers all the bases. "May you be healed. May you be blessed. May you have peace." I figure everyone I know could do with a little more healing, blessings, and peace. And by the time I've prayed for friends, neighbors, colleagues, pets, foreign countries, writers, movie stars, and politicians, I'm asleep—or it's time to get up.

So let me just say here, many thanks for your love and support. I'm happy to pray for you all.

Love and Hugs,
Debra

Global Warming

A hot flash is not like being in an overheated room or sitting in the sun. Nor is it a flash, like lightening, over in a split second. Believe me, that would be preferable. This is how it is at night: I am suddenly awake. Not the kind of startled awake from a sudden sound where your heart is pounding and you're listening hard. No, I am suddenly awake as if I were in the middle of a job interview, my mind totally engaged and alert.

I think, "Hmm, why am I awake? Oh, yeah, I'm about to have a hot flash. But first—the cold flash!" A wave of goose bumps travels from my ankles all the way up to my scalp culminating in a giant shiver. Then pressure builds in my skull and radiates to my face. My ears start burning and turn bright red. It's a miracle my hair doesn't go up in flames.

My core feels as if there is a nuclear bomb going off, which makes my chest, stomach, and back heat up to approximately 350 degrees Fahrenheit. You can easily melt cheese slices on my belly. My crotch feels as if someone has planted a Bunsen burner between my legs. Then I start sweating like Seabiscuit coming down the stretch. Impressive really.

Over a period of two weeks I went from thinking "How fascinating" to "This sucks!" and then back to "How fascinating." Getting mad was no good, because it kept me awake longer.

I sought advice from one of my patients.

"The moment you wake up, get up and pee. That way you are already out of that hot bed when the heat comes on. Of course it helps tremendously to be bald. Getting your head cool is paramount." She gave me a pitying look. "But you have all that *hair*."

It was the first time anyone ever felt sorry for me for not losing all my hair.

I had never in my life had insomnia—not really. A sleepless night here and there, but this was different. Night after night of being awake three to four hours. Plenty of time to go over my entire life and reflect on how things were or how I thought they should be. Which brings me to my family of origin.

Letting People off My Hook

When my sister visited just after my surgery, the three of us went to see the movie *Millions*. In it there is a scene where the little boy is talking to his dead mother. She says to him, "Have faith in people. It makes them strong."

I took that as a sign from Mr. Martha Miyagi to have faith my sister and my parents would reconcile. "Have faith in Lynie," I told myself. "It will make her strong. Have faith in Mom and Dad. It will make them strong."

It was important to me before, but now it felt absolutely essential that my family be intact. Why is this? When you get cancer you very quickly learn the important things in life are not things at all, but relationships. The job, the car, the house, and everything in it are nothing compared to who will come and hold your hand. Who will listen to you? Who will bring you soup?

My relationships were precious to me, especially my family, and I wanted everyone to be together.

I had hoped my mom's cancer diagnosis and then my diagnosis would somehow heal the estrangement between my parents and my sister. It seemed like perfect timing because everyone was feeling vulnerable and emotional, and I was sure everything would be forgiven. I couldn't be with my mom for her surgery, so one scenario was my Dad would call Lynie and ask her to come down and be with them. My other dream was that Lynie would call them and say, "Mom and Dad, let's just forget the past. I'm here for you now."

But my perfect little scene was complicated by the fact that Paul, Lynie's son, had an emergency appendectomy. Who should she be with: her seventeen-year-old son, her sister having a mastectomy, or her mother who she hadn't been close to in sixteen years? Of course she chose her son. I would have, too.

Often a life-threatening illness brings people back together. I was talking to a young woman whose mother was coming in for chemotherapy. The daughter was seventeen, very bright, and her mother had had breast cancer since Kaylie was ten. Her parents divorced before she was born.

"It was always a big tense thing with my parents, me going back and forth. My mom would get mad, and then my dad would get mad. But when my mom was diagnosed, everything changed overnight. It was totally weird."

"What do you mean?" I asked.

"Well, it used to be if one of them wanted me for an extra day it was a 'concession.' That's all I heard from both of them, 'I'm making so many concessions to your mother,' or 'to your father.' And then when mom got cancer, it was no longer a concession. It was just the way we did things. Everybody just chilled. They were both more relaxed with each other."

"How do you explain that?" I thought perhaps she could let me in on the secret.

"I think they finally got that life is short, and they were being stupid. I mean, they did really love each other at some point, and I think they remembered that."

I had seen this kind of thing happen when I worked in hospice. Children who have been estranged for years find out their parent is dying, and they suddenly show up. They get reacquainted with their parent and find to their amazement they actually like them after all. The reconciliation is joyful but also bittersweet.

That is what I wanted for my family: a joyful but bittersweet reunion. So while I lay awake at night after a hot flash, I would think about this and pray. Well, I'm not really sure if this was prayer or just plain fantasizing.

I saw us having Thanksgiving dinner together at Lynie's house. My parents had never seen her house. I thought maybe being on her home turf would be more comfortable for Lynie than returning to our ancestral ranch-style house in the Silicon Valley. Besides, she had a bigger dining room.

There we would be cooking in the kitchen, my mom, my sister, and I. The men would be watching football in the living room—except Wes would keep coming in to see if we needed any help because that's the kind of guy he is. My niece would be late because she always is. My nephew would be watching the game too, but quietly because he is a man of few words.

We'd all be jolly in the kitchen, sipping champagne between chopping onions and toasting pecans. Lynie would run out and look at the TV every so often because she is a big football fan. The guys would be cheering in the living room, and we women would start to get a little tense wondering if some people were drinking too much champagne.

But we'd keep on chopping and toasting, and then Mom would say, "I don't chop like that. I chop like *this*." Lynie and I would exchange looks, and things would get a little tenser.

Then there would be a roar from the living room, and Dad would be bellowing at the defense or the coach or the quarterback. Wes and my brother-in-law, Dan, would be calming him down. Then Wes would come in the kitchen and beg to do the dishes, and we would all feel even tenser and decide that no one was getting any more champagne, and maybe we shouldn't have wine with dinner. Then there would be an argument about who was being a hard head and who was not.

When I got to that point in my prayer/fantasy I'd move on to the next holiday.

The problem was that I ran out of holidays, and I came to the realization that families are complicated and crazy and sometimes unlikable, but that's what families are. No matter how much I fantasized, it was never going to be perfect.

All those photos in *Sunset* magazine of families cooking together don't show the teenage daughter flipping off her mother. They don't explain the reason the father has a shaved head is because he's thinking of leaving his family and becoming a Buddhist monk. They don't show the aunt using her inhaler because she's allergic to the gorgeous Bernese mountain dog in the photo who not only has worms, but regularly humps the Barcalounger.

No, families aren't perfect and neither is life, or why would I be lying awake from a chemo-induced hot flash?

After several nights of this I was a wreck. My sister called one afternoon not knowing what a mental case I was. So when she innocently asked me how I was feeling, I answered, "I'm so sad you and Mom and Dad still don't speak, and I'm afraid they're going to die, and it will be too late. I hoped having cancer would make you see how important family is, and they're your parents and they're sad, too. I don't want to have to *die* to make you see that."

I said all that in one breath, but I was crying at the end. There was a big pause and then Lynie said, "It sounds like you're having a bad day."

She was right about that. She was also correct in realizing I was making my sadness her problem. It wasn't. It was my problem. I'd fallen into that whole trap of, "If only X would do Y, then I'd be happy."

She was also smart not to engage me in this conversation. In the past we'd try to talk about it, and she'd said different things like, "I'll take that under consideration," which is like taking the

Watchtower from the Jehovah's Witnesses and throwing it in the recycling bin while they're watching. One time she said, "It's not up to you."

It was the one subject we couldn't talk about. I had both a burning desire and absolute fear of bringing it up. I love my sister like no other, and I didn't want to do anything that would jeopardize our relationship. But not talking about it created a distance between us. I wondered if there would ever be a step toward reconciliation, and who would take it.

The thing that made it hard for me was in recent years, Wes and I really did have fun with my parents. They didn't drive me crazy like they used to. They had changed, but so had we. I no longer made them drink Peet's coffee when they visited. I brewed Yuban. When we visited, they brewed Yuban really strong for us and diluted theirs. They hadn't achieved perfection or anything— my God, my dad is still a Republican, and Mom adores the paintings of Thomas Kinkade.

I consulted Jesus about this. He's really such a hippie. All I heard from him was, "Love them and chill out."

Searching scripture for Jesus's behavior toward his own parents, I came up with him being rude to his mother at a wedding. She tells him the hosts have run out of wine. Different translations have him saying, "What have I to do with thee?" "What has that to do with us?" "Why do you involve me?" In other words, "Why are you telling me?" As if she had said, "Oy vey, Jesus, here we are with no wine. Do something!"

What about the Ten Commandments? "Thou shalt honor thy father and thy mother." My sister is a Christian, but I knew that quoting scripture to her wouldn't make her do what I wanted.

I consulted Gloria, one of my long-time patients. She had been living with cancer for fifteen years. She also had a son who didn't speak to her.

"Debra," she said. "You pray about this, and then you let it go, my darling. You can no more make people do what you want than God can make us do what He wants. We're provided the opportunity, that's all. I've apologized to my son, but he just can't forgive me."

"But you're his *mom*."

"I know that!" she said impatiently. "But I can't make him forgive me. You're being thick-headed here. Just because you have cancer doesn't mean you get everything your way."

"I know."

"Do you?"

"It's worked well for other things."

"Well, it's not going to work for this. And you'd be wise to stop spreading that 'do I have to die?' manure."

I hated that she was right.

Wedding Break

As the months went by I bagged out on more social plans because I was just too tired. But I had made one I had no intention of breaking, for it is a rare and wonderful thing for a babysitter to officiate at the wedding of a babysittee.

In my last two years at UC Berkeley, my girlfriends and I moved up into the Berkeley hills to live in the house of a professor on sabbatical. We had no idea we had moved into a neighborhood of young families. All we cared about was that the rent was a good deal and the view was gorgeous. All the neighbors cared about was that we were five female college students—babysitter jackpot!

My friends and I moved in one morning and by that afternoon, two people had already knocked on our door to ask if we could babysit that weekend. They had that crazed, desperate look in their eyes I would later come to recognize in my own friends.

The Thomsons were my favorite customers because: (1) they had a pool, (2) they had a grand piano, (3) they had a dog (a cairn terrier like Max), (4) they had Peet's coffee, (5) they had a great view of San Francisco, and most importantly, (6) they had three great kids, Heather, Colin, and Alison.

Colin was the soloist at our wedding and now twenty years later, I was the minister at his. The entire family was very sweet and said they understood if I couldn't come because I was on chemo. But there was no way I was going to miss this.

We flew down to Berkeley on the weekend, and the wedding was held on a Monday. This is traditionally the dark night at the theater, and because Colin and Karen are both actors and singers, as were many of their friends, this was a sensible thing to do. It was also great for me because I got chemo on Thursday, and I was just starting to perk up on Monday.

I had forgotten how Berkeley could be cool and cloudy in the morning, and then the sun breaks out around 11 a.m. and it's glorious. We hiked up the Strawberry Canyon Fire Trail and walked in Tilden Park. The change of scenery recharged me. Even the air was different, drier and smelling of eucalyptus. I realized in the six weeks I'd been on chemo, I'd allowed my life to become mostly work and chemo. This trip reminded me there is more life out there, and other people are having big important things happen to them—like getting married.

The wedding was held outside of the Brazil Room in Tilden Park. We stood under an arch made of twigs and flowers and a huge green lawn spread out behind us to the edge of the woods. Colin's family is Scottish, so there was a bagpiper and lots of men running around in kilts. Colin wore a dress kilt. Karen was gorgeous in a magnificent red taffeta gown—very *Gone with the Wind*-y.

I really do make the homily as personal as I can, and because they were actors, I talked about scripts. We all have different scripts in our heads about lots of things: marriage, children, death. These scripts are based on what we've seen or what we've read or what we're told. We don't realize we can script our lives any way we want.

This is what I told Karen and Colin. "Just know you two can write your own script and make your marriage be any way you want it to be. And know you can rewrite it at any time you like."

As I was writing their homily, I realized I felt the same way about my cancer experience. There are a lot of books and movies out there about the horror and anguish of cancer and chemo. I wanted to do it with more humor and less drama, while at the same time being real. You can't control what life gives you, but you can choose your response. That means you don't have to follow anyone's script but your own.

Speaking of which, I always give the couple a wedding blessing, which is not something you find in all ceremonies. The one I chose for Colin and Karen was the Apache Wedding Blessing. I asked them to join their hands together, and then I wrapped their hands with the ends of my stole. Then I put my hands around theirs. I call this the "hand sandwich," and I make this little joke to myself to keep from crying.

It is this particular moment in the ceremony where I am always fighting back tears. Perhaps it is because the three of us are standing so close together, and I'm sucking up some of that love they feel for one another. Or maybe it's the paradox of having an intimate private moment between the couple and me be so undeniably public. I always feel overwhelmed at the honor of giving a wedding blessing, so perhaps that's the reason I choke up.

But this time I knew I was near tears because I looked at Wes sitting in the front row and thought, "You were marvelous through the 'for better' and 'in health' part. And you're astonishing in this 'for worse' and 'in sickness' phase."

So we stood there with our hands together, and I took a moment to clear my throat, which gave my mind time to say, "Hand sandwich. Ha-ha! Hand sandwich!"

I smiled and looked up at them and said, "Now you will feel no rain for the two of you will be shelter to the other. Now you will feel no cold for each of you will be warmth to the other. Now there is no more loneliness, but you are two persons with one life before you. Go now to your dwelling-place to enter into the days of your togetherness, and may your days be good and long upon the earth."

The congregation reacts differently to this blessing depending on the situation. In Seattle the first line gets the crowd stirring. At a freezing outdoor ceremony or a winter wedding, it's the second line. Colin and Karen had been living in togetherness for some time and had already bought and remodeled their dwelling-place together. It seemed to me that everyone sighed on the last line: "And may your days be good and long upon the earth."

Meltdown Moment

"Hey—wait a minute!" I said aloud when I saw the posted flyer about the staff support group, "Caring for Our Own." How could there be a support group without me knowing about it? Shouldn't *I* be leading the group?

I felt like a kid who just found out her parents were in therapy because of their unruly child. I knew it wasn't just about me, but also about my co-worker who was receiving treatment. And in fact, it wasn't really about either of us, but was about how the staff felt about caring for us.

The ugly head of role and identity issues reared up and bit me right on the ass. *I* wanted to facilitate the support group! I was a chaplain. I was tired of being a patient. My feelings regressed all the way to "I don't want to eat my vegetables! I want candy!"

This was my state of mind when I turned the corner around nursing station A/B, just before my infusion, and one of the nurses sang out, "Welcome, Debra!"

"What?"

"You're one of our patients and I'm welcoming you!" Any other day and I would have laughed and smiled, but I had transmogrified into a four-year-old. Like any good four-year-old worth her salt I started crying. And even as I said the words, "I don't want to do this anymore!" I realized I was not even halfway through my chemo. The nurses all looked horrified, which compounded my misery because I was making them feel bad. Ping-pong suffering!

I stood there unable to move. One of the nurses came up, put her arm around me, and walked me to my bed. I don't mean she had her arm resting gently upon my shoulders. No. She was literally pushing me down the hall.

When I got to my room I got into bed, and the nurses brought me warm blankets.

"How about a little Ativan?" one of them asked. (Ativan is the pharmaceutical equivalent of hot milk and graham crackers.)

I nodded still sniffing and blowing my nose. This was not in my script. What about "more humor, less drama"? What about "grace and charm"? I forgot about holding things "lightly and gently," which means deviating from the script or the plan is no big deal.

Now if any other patient were behaving like this, one of the nurses would have come and found me. She probably would say something like "The patient in room 31 is just having a hard time, really tearful. Could you go in and talk with her?"

So who could be the chaplain to me? My boss had asked me if I wanted a chaplain and I said no. My department was small—four people including me. We didn't see one another much because we each had our separate caseloads and worked in different buildings. I thought it would be weird to suddenly start confiding in one of them just because I had cancer.

So while I waited for my lab results and before Wes got there, I thought about what I would say to myself as my own chaplain.

"Hey, nice shoes," said my chaplain self with a big grin.

"Half price. Macy's."

"Sweet. So how are you doing? You look a little verklempt."

"Oh, I'm just a little freaked out because nobody told me about this staff support group."

"Sounds like they must care about you a lot, if they need a support group about giving you care. That's a happy problem."

"Yeah."

"If you were facilitating the group how would you handle it?"

I thought for a moment before answering myself. "I wouldn't go running to the employee/patient and say, 'We're doing a support group because of you.' I'd probably just quietly let the staff know about the group."

"Would you keep it a secret?"

"No! That would be so creepy!"

"No kidding. So you would pretty much handle it the way they've handled it."

"Um, yeah."

"Cool. What else is going on with you?"

"Most of the time I'm okay. But today, my implant is hurting and I'm nauseous and tired because I haven't been sleeping. I'm trying to be a good soldier."

"Since when are you a fan of the military?"

"Since never."

"How about if you just feel your feelings and then move on from there?"

"Okay, so I feel sad and depressed and sick and whiny and shitty and my chemo stretches out before me like a cross-country drive from Seattle to Miami. I miss my old strong and healthy self, and I'm afraid it's only going to get worse because of the cumulative effects of this chemo."

My chaplain self nodded sympathetically. "It's good to name all the feelings. Makes everything a little more manageable. And don't forget to tell your nurse you're not sleeping."

"I'm feeling pretty sleepy right now."

"That's the Ativan."

"Would you pray with me before you go—the kind of prayer with words you say with other patients?"

"Sure." I reach over and hold my hand. "Ground of Our Being, we can't pretend to understand everything you allow in our lives, but we do know you are with us in every moment of every night and every day. We pray now you would lay your healing hand upon Debra, help her to relax into your care. We pray for both Debra and Wes that you would keep their hearts open to your spirit of peace and comfort and love and strength. And we pray all would be blessed, all would be healed, and all would have peace. Amen."

I would have said amen, but I was asleep.

Breast-fed

There was nothing like losing my breast and getting chemo to give me street cred with the patients. My treatment experience was turning out to be pretty useful for many reasons. One is that I was walking proof you could be on CMF and have a life. This was particularly important for first time patients. The nurses often pointed at a room and said, "First time CMF. Pretty scared."

"Say no more." Then I'd waltz in there and let them know I was on the same stuff! When I shared this information every single CMF patient was so relieved. There's just nothing like talking with someone who is going, or has gone through it.

Then there was the matter of the replacement part. First you should know the nurses always asked me first if they could tell their patients about my treatment. I always said yes. One day I was asked to talk with a young woman from Alaska who had questions about reconstruction.

We chatted a bit about the weather in Alaska, and we talked about the cute little crocheted cap that covered her bald head. Then she lowered her voice and said, "My nurse told me you had breast reconstruction—an implant. Will you tell me about it?"

"Oh, sure," I said. I recounted my whole experience even including the phrase, "hurt like hell." She lapped up every word, starving as she was for information.

"Wow," she said. "Thanks for being so honest and open about it. You know I'm not from here, and I don't have anybody I can ask about this." She paused and then leaned forward. "Would you show it to me?"

"What?!"

"Your breast. Could I—see it?"

This was the moment, some would later say, that I should have referred her to a support group or a cancer hotline, or an Internet site on breast reconstruction. But they weren't there in that moment, watching her bite her lip and twist the corners of the blankets. They weren't looking at her beautiful young face as she was wondering if she would ever again be an attractive woman. They didn't see the pleading look in her eyes or hear how hard it was for her to ask.

I said, "Sure."

I was wearing a long dress that had neither buttons down the front nor a zipper up the back. I had no choice but to hike it up over my shoulders, so I was in nothing but my underwear. I hoped nobody would come bursting through the curtain catching the chaplain half-naked with a patient.

She looked at my breast critically for a few moments and then stretched her hand out toward me. "May I touch it?"

I thought, "Well, I've gone this far." I realized it's exactly this kind of thinking that causes young women to lose their virginity.

"Yes," I said.

Twenty years of ministering to the spiritual needs of the sick and dying. Three years of seminary, an internship in the parish, an internship in the hospital, board certification, and my whole ministry had come to this: letting a stranger touch my breast. The irony and the wonder of it took my breath away.

I looked up at her and her eyes were shining with tears. "Thank you," she whispered.

And suddenly it all came flashing back to me—the scripture I chose for my ordination. It was from the book of Isaiah, where God asks, "Whom shall I send?" And the prophet Isaiah answers, "Here am I. Send me!"

But, of course, there was nothing in my ordination or any of my training about exactly what I'd be sent to do. But then that's my task: to be open to serving in even the most bizarre ways. I think if Mr. Martha Miyagi supplied us with a list of all the ways we will be called to serve, we'd never sign up. What if at my ordination I received a list that included "get breast cancer, have mastectomy, receive chemo, and show a reconstructed breast"? Better we should figure it out as we go along.

After she was done examining my breast, and I settled back into my clothes, we talked a little more, comparing notes on chemo and nausea. When I stood to leave she said, "I'm so glad you came by. There's nobody else I could talk with about this."

"Well, I was sent," I said.

"Oh, you mean by my nurse."

"Yes," I said. Because I believe God speaks through nurses all the time.

That's the funny part about being a chaplain: everyone thinks I've got the Holy Spirit on my speed dial. The staff will say things like "Would you put in a word for me with God? You've got a better connection." But I watch the Spirit using their hands and using their words all the time.

Often the medical staff will tip-toe in to check a chemo pump, and they'll be all apologetic and I'll sometimes think, "Well, if you had known we were talking about SpongeBob SquarePants you wouldn't have been so respectful."

But I don't mention it.

However, I do encourage the medical staff to talk with their patients about spiritual issues. When patients ask their nurse or doctor, "Do you think there's a God?" this is not the time to run out and call the chaplain. They are asking *that* person in *that* moment. It's like being in a restaurant when you are just about ready to start your meal and you see something unrecognizable in your soup. A busboy walks by and you ask, "Excuse me, but is this a *fly* in my soup?"

You don't want him to reply, "Oh, let me get your waiter." The busboy is right there. You're asking *him*. You don't have to be a waiter to recognize a fly. You don't have to be a chaplain to discuss spirituality.

So I urge staff to relax and share their spiritual beliefs for a few minutes. Of course, this doesn't work the other way. I can't be a doctor for a few minutes—although I have been known to give advice on constipation.

Seven

A WHITE BLOOD CELL CHRISTMAS

Dear Fabulous Family and Friends,

Santa has already come to the Jarvis–Van Voorhis family. I'm finishing chemo three weeks early. Woo-hoo! My last infusion is December 8, the day after our twentieth anniversary! Woo-hoo-hoo!

My oncologist suggested stopping after pointing out my white blood cells were deeply unhappy. Most of them had packed their bags and left for Florida, and the ones that were still here were protesting and threatening to leave.

I am thrilled and look forward to once again being able to eat chocolate and drink wine. But I have some positive things to say about chemo. Because I used to hate them, we had a backlog of those tart herbal teas with names like, "Zesty Grape Spittle," "Corrosive Cranberry," and "Acid Berry Sting." But now I love, love, love them. I crave sour things, and I crave salty things. The clerks at Whole Foods had to pull me away from the deli after they found me face down in the Kalamata olives. I have lemon sorbet for breakfast. I sneak shots of balsamic vinegar. I dream of lime-flavored tortilla chips.

So hopefully I will get my normal taste back, but I will not get my estrogen back and boy, do I miss it. To counter the hot flashes, I was put on a low dose of Effexor. It was magic! Hot flashes gone!

A few weeks after being on Effexor, my mother visited me. I complained about blurry vision and she said, "Honey, you're just getting old. You'll have to wear glasses now." I was so comforted. I took her to the airport and put her in the wrong line, *not* because of the "getting old" remark, but because I couldn't see the airport signs!

Depressed, I came home, looked in the mirror, and said, "You're getting old—and why are your eyes totally dilated!?" The next day one of my colleagues looked up Effexor and w-a-a-a-y down on the bottom of the list of side effects was "excessive pupil dilation." Wes thought I looked sexy with my dilated eyes. I couldn't see a thing and told him he looked sexy, too.

So now I'm on a combination of meds that are not quite as effective. When I wake up and wave the blankets up and down to cool off, Wes always partially awakens and asks, "Wha-a-a-?"

I whisper, "Darling, you've won the Nobel Prize in medicine." He then goes back to sleep and always wakes up in a good mood.

The replacement part seems to be slowly dropping, like the lighted ball in Times Square. I can only hope I don't find it on my hipbone on New Year's Eve. But I'm grateful for so many other things: the great care I received at the SCCA, my mensch of a husband, the fact that although I lost some hair, I still have most of it. In fact, I am going to grow it even longer and then cut it off and donate it. I thought it might be kind of cool for someone with cancer to have a wig made with survivor hair. So my hairdresser is just trimming it and coaching me on how not to look like an aging hippie.

Someone said to me, "This cancer must be like Hurricane Katrina in your life." Well, sort of. But where Katrina exposed corruption, deceit, and neglect, cancer in my life has exposed overwhelming love, care, and support. Now here is where I'm supposed to say what I've learned and what I'll change in my life. But here's the thing: Going through treatment is a lot like walking on a rope bridge. You're so intent on getting to the other side, you have no idea over what you have just crossed.

Or to switch metaphors, I've been in a deep mine for six months and have been digging my way out. When I emerge I'll take some time to look in my bag and see what nuggets I've brought out. Some will be just rocks. But some will be gold. I'll let you know.

Love and Hugs,
Debra

Promise Breaker

I let three months elapse between e-mail updates because I was in the daily grind of treatment. I worked at the clinic Tuesday, Wednesday, and Thursday. I received chemo on Thursday afternoon. I recovered Friday, Saturday, Sunday, and Monday. There was really nothing new to report. Just trying to get through.

I continued walking the Deer Loop throughout the summer and fall. Amy asked Max's owner again if he would give him or sell him to us, but again he said no. Like many cairn terriers, Max was wild about chasing a tennis ball. So I went over and threw the ball for him every day.

So here I was halfway through my chemo, feeling a bit down, and generally mentally addled. I missed my brain. Chemo brain is a very real thing. It's not just going into a room and forgetting what you came in for. It's also forgetting words, people's names, and who said what when. I started getting one patient's story mixed up with another's.

I'd lean forward and say something to a patient like, "Last week you talked about how Pixie's death made you think about the meaning of your own life. Do you have any more thoughts on that?" And they'd give me a blank look and I'd go, "Oh, wasn't her name Pixie?"

"Who's Pixie?"

"Your poodle."

"I don't have a poodle. I have a shepherd mix named Larry."

"Oh, I'm so sorry!"

Then I'd visit my next patient and say, "Mr. Shepherd, how are you?"

"I'm not Mr. Shepherd."

"Uh, right. Larry?"

Quality pastoral care.

Chemo brain makes you feel as if half your neurons are not on duty, but instead are sitting around smoking cigarettes and sipping martinis. It was nothing like the pleasant buzz I got from a glass of wine. It was more like the feeling I got in high school math class when the teacher would explain something to me, and I'd wonder why he was speaking Swahili. I'd nod and look at the numbers on the page, but would have no idea what he was talking about.

So I was in this befuddled state of mind just before our annual Labor Day trip to the beach at Iron Springs. We had been going there for fifteen years, the main reason being they accepted dogs. But even after our lab/dalmatian mix Cokey died, we continued to go. And now I had an overwhelming desire to have a dog at the beach. Specifically, Max. I ran this idea by Wes. He wasn't enthused.

"It will just be a hassle and his owner will never let him go."

Perhaps it was my daily association with Max that caused me to hang on to this idea with the tenacity of a terrier. We *had* to take Max to the beach.

The day before we left I knew I had to act. I drove directly to Max's house after work. This meant I was still in my work clothes, so I looked pretty upstanding and responsible.

As usual Max was in the front yard and was delighted to see me. I threw the ball for him a few times before I walked up to the door and knocked.

His owner answered the door. He was wearing shorts and no shirt and was pale and skinny.

"Hi, I'm the woman who comes over and plays with Max. And I know this will sound really crazy, but my husband and I are going to the beach for five days and I'm wondering if we can take him. A little beach vacation for your dog."

His eyes widened and he actually took a step back from me as if I were a deranged bag lady.

I felt desperate. I must have Max! I played the cancer card. "And since my *mastectomy*, and during all this time I've been on *chemo* Max has been such a big part of my healing." He still said nothing and just stood there looking at me.

"Well, think about it," I said lamely.

"Let me talk to my wife."

"Oh, okay!" I hastily scribbled my home phone on one of my business cards. "Here's my number!" I hoped knowing that I worked at a big international cancer center would convince this man I could take care of his dog. I drove home whooping in the car.

He called an hour later and said, "Okay, you can take him." I was shocked, but then why would he mind? Max stayed out all day and all night.

"Anything that moves, he'll bolt," he said. "So promise me you'll keep him on the leash at all times."

"I promise." My heart sank because that is the beauty of Iron Springs: the gigantic off-leash beach.

"And if you want him to do his business, just say, 'Do your business!' And if you say it sort of loud, then he'll do it."

I wanted to ask, "Does Max have business *cards?*" but I didn't want to screw up the deal.

We picked him up Thursday afternoon after my chemo. All they gave us was Max, his crate (with no blanket in it!), a ball, his leash, and some food. No soft bed. No other toys. I thought about what we would send with Cokey: her bed, her toys, her leash, her treats, her homemade food, and a five-page instruction sheet. So maybe we were a little over-protective. Some would say neurotic.

Unfortunately my brain was badly scrambled after chemo. Honestly, I don't know if it was psychological or physical or emotional. I forgot the napkins, the paper towels, the coffee canisters (which I had filled the night before), our latte mugs, our tea mugs, and enough bedtime tea. I left a carton of milk on the kitchen counter. But who cared? We had a dog!

However it was eighty degrees in Seattle, and our car chose this day to have the heater stuck on the *on* position. Nothing we did could fix it. Wes had a headache, I was feeling sick, and Max was panting in the back. We rolled down all the windows but the noise and stink from the big trucks was unbearable.

After four hours of this torture, we arrived at Iron Springs just before sunset. As soon as the three of us got on the beach, I knew when I died, I'd be shot straight to Hell because I kept Max on the leash for about two minutes, then let him go. I broke my promise.

But have you ever seen a cairn terrier chasing sandpipers at sunset?

He went after them in earnest with the kind of joy found in knowing your life's purpose. All the hair on his face and body blew straight back so he looked like a streaking comet. Every once in a while Max would look back at us as if to say, "I'm doing my best to catch them and thanks for giving me the job." He was a bullet whizzing through a cloud of birds against a pink-orange sky.

It was breathtaking, staggering, hilarious. Both of us were laughing and crying and forgot all about the car, the headache, chemo, and cancer.

Yes, I broke my promise.

But all I heard was, *You are forgiven.*

To See for Herself

A few weeks after our trip to the beach, my mom came for a visit. As I said before, the imagination can be worse than the reality, so I wanted her to come to chemo with Wes and me and to see what happened. I also wanted her to see I was not an emaciated wreck dragging myself to work.

As soon as I got her home and hung up her coat, I sat her down on the bed. "Let's do the boob show, Mom." I wanted to see her lumpectomy and wanted to show her my implant. She lifted up her blouse and unhooked her bra. There was just a small divot in her breast and then a scar under her arm where she had some nodes removed.

I lifted up my sweater and she gasped. "Is that a tumor?" She was looking at my port.

"No, no! That's where they put the chemo in. What do you think of my breast?" I could see her eyes well up.

"It looks good, honey."

She came to chemo with me a few days later. She had a nervous pinched look on her face. I introduced her to everyone as we walked through the infusion suite, and she seemed to relax a little. But once we got into my room, she sat in a chair between my bed and the wall, never took off her coat, folded her arms over her chest, made herself as small as possible, and watched the Food Network. Every now and then she would look over at me when Sherry was doing something like taking my blood pressure or accessing my port. She witnessed the whole procedure through glances.

Sherry brought me warm blankets and cookies. "See, Mom? See how they take such good care of me?"

I wondered if this brought back memories of my illness when I was an infant. Just before my mastectomy, I was talking to my dad and he said, "Sweetie, you were on that table as a baby and fifty years later you are on that table again." Then he broke down crying. So I was sure this wasn't easy for Mom, but she didn't say anything.

As usual the weekend was a low point for me physically. I wanted to take Mom to my favorite fabric store, to the bead shop, and to a clothing outlet, but I couldn't get off the couch. She was sitting on the couch with me reading a cookbook when I laid my head in her lap.

"Mom, I'm so sorry, I think I'm too tired to go out."

She breathed an unmistakable sigh of relief and said, "For once our energy levels are the same."

Early Parole

I couldn't keep my white blood cell count up so my oncologist would hold my chemo. The next week the count would be back up, I'd receive chemo, and then it would plummet again. I'd miss chemo, it would rise, I'd get chemo, counts would fall ad nauseam, and I do mean *nauseam*.

My oncologist thought this was crazy, as I was already on what she called a "homeopathic dose" of chemo. Chemo kills rapidly proliferating cells like my white blood cells, so if there were are any cancer cells hanging around, which proliferate even faster, they were surely gone by now.

I've known patients who felt very vulnerable and very afraid about stopping early. I didn't feel that way. Deep down I felt this was the right thing for my body. It had gotten to the point where the cumulative effect of the chemo was overwhelming my body. I felt crumbly around the edges like the last cookie in the bag.

Having cancer messes not just with how you look, but with how you think of yourself. I've never thought of myself as a delicate flower, more like a strong, sturdy dandelion. But here I was tired, weak, with wimpy white cells, peeling fingernails, and Effexor-dilated eyes.

My patient Gloria said to me, "Get over it! It has nothing to do with your moral fiber. It is not an ethical dilemma. These are side effects, not personality flaws."

So I decided to continue to think of myself as a sturdy dandelion that was not cut down by the mower, but temporarily flattened.

Great Lengths

I hadn't seen Rita since the beginning of my chemo, and she was in the clinic to receive her quarterly dose of Zometa, a bone-building drug that also prevents bone metastases. I knocked and stepped into her bay with a big smile on my face. She had a big smile, too, which promptly turned into a surprised frown.

"You didn't lose your hair!" she wailed.

"Good to see you too."

"C'mere, is that really your hair?'

I sat down next to her chair and she pulled on my hair. "Hmph. You must be on the Barbie chemo. Chemo-lite."

I would have been furious, but honestly, I was too tired. And it wasn't like I hadn't heard this before. I gave Rita my standard line. "I've lost about a fourth of it, but I had lots to begin with."

There is a hierarchy of suffering in the breast cancer world. The variables are surgery, chemo, radiation, and total hair loss. I realize total hair loss is a side effect and not a treatment, but it is a major variable.

So the most sympathy goes to those who have had a double mastectomy, chemo, radiation, and total hair loss. At the bottom is a lumpectomy only.

Hair loss trumps surgery, radiation trumps chemo. So even though I had surgery and chemo, because I didn't lose my hair, I was down at the bottom. I didn't really care because my friends and colleagues were supportive anyway. But I've talked with patients on CMF who stopped going to support groups because they felt so apologetic. They felt as if their situation wasn't bad enough to warrant support.

"We need our own support group," a patient said to me. "Because those of us on CMF have all these pissy little problems but we still look pretty good."

Even more unhappy are women with DCIS. "I had someone tell me it's not really cancer!" a woman said to me.

"Of course it's cancer," I said. "It just means the cancer, the carcinoma, is still in your ducts. You know, the car hasn't left the garage and driven down the highway. But there's still a *car* in there." I was pretty proud of this analogy, especially since "car" sounds like carcinoma, but I could see my laser-like wit was lost on her.

I don't know what it is that makes us competitive in our suffering. "You think *that's* bad? Well, listen to *this*." Is it one-upmanship? Is it ego? Is it a bid for attention?

I've even had a patient say, "There's a woman in my support group who I think is enjoying her cancer a little too much." Enjoying cancer? I did not understand this.

Then one night, Wes and I were in a restaurant when a bald woman came in and sat down at a table with her friends. She spoke loudly and sounded as if she was boasting to everyone in the place.

"When I went for my *chemotherapy* last week, my *oncologist* was worried I might get an *infection*. So my nurse gave me a *shot in my belly* to stimulate my *white blood cells*." Her friends were cooing in sympathy and patting her arm and squeezing her hand.

I could see how someone might think, "She's enjoying this a *little* too much." But to me her voice sounded hollow and filled with need. Did it take cancer for her to get this kind of loving attention from her friends?

The waitress brought our meals, and as we held hands for a moment of silent gratitude, I said a quick prayer for her healing—both physically and emotionally.

Promise Keeper

I loved Kari. She was one of the few patients who actually wanted to talk theology and Biblical history with me. But that's not why

I loved her. I loved her because she struggled with her faith, she asked questions, and she dared to reject some beliefs.

"What do you think Jesus meant by this?" she'd ask. "Why was the Old Testament God so mean? Do you believe people who aren't Christians are going to Hell?"

I let her know the correct term was "Hebrew scriptures," not "Old Testament." It's not old to Jews, only to Christians because we're comparing it to the New Testament, which is correctly called the "Christian scriptures."

I felt like quite the mentor when I told her that or when I brought her books I read in seminary. But I felt like her teenage best friend when I brought in Christopher Moore's hilarious novel *Lamb* about what Jesus did between the ages of thirteen and thirty-five. I handed it to her in a brown paper bag and said, "If anyone asks, you didn't get this from me." She loved it.

We had the kind of easy friendship that comes from meeting every week, which unfortunately we did. I mean it was unfortunate because we were meeting at a cancer center.

"How do you hear God?" she asked me one day. I told her about Mr. Martha Miyagi. I even told her about the cedar tree in the fence. She said God often spoke to her through her children.

"One day I was holding Peter on my lap and I started yelling at his brother who was spilling Cheerios all over the floor. And Peter reached up and stroked my face and said, 'Be nice, Mommy.'"

A few weeks after I was diagnosed, she said to me, "I left a gift for you on your desk that I think you'll find helpful." I returned to my desk to find a white baseball cap with the word "Cancer" embroidered on it. There was a little pink bow taped crookedly on the front and when I pulled off the bow I realized why it had been placed off-center. Underneath the bow was the embroidered word, "Fuck." Fuck Cancer.

You may think everyone with cancer is a "cancer victim," but that is not true. Kari was a "person with cancer." She was doing her best to live her life and treat her disease. She wasn't able to do everything she wanted to do, because she was so often fatigued and nauseous, but she was never a victim.

We even discussed that term. "Victim makes you sound like some kind of suffering prey," she said.

"Yes," I said, "like 'the gazelle was a victim of the lion.' But I don't feel like prey—just horribly inconvenienced."

"Yes," she said. "Cancer is terribly annoying."

Even though her disease progressed, her doctor always had some new experimental chemo up his sleeve, so she wasn't discouraged.

She had been dealing with breast cancer for three years. She was only thirty-four and had been diagnosed with a Stage IV cancer. She attended a conservative evangelical church.

"But I don't really agree with them," she confessed. "I don't believe you'll go to Hell if you don't love Jesus. There's lots of other stuff I don't believe in."

"Then why do you keep going?"

She looked sheepish. "Because the women there are all so nice and help so much with the kids." She had three little boys.

I nodded silently. Childcare is a big deal when your husband works full time and you are coming in for chemo every week. Then there are the scans, the doctor visits, the extra visits when you need IV hydration.

"The women have become my friends, but I'm afraid to say what I really think when they talk about God."

"So what do you do?"

"I go to the bathroom."

She wasn't afraid to talk about death, though.

"I do think there is some kind of reunion with loved ones," she said. "I'm looking forward to seeing my dad." Her father died of cancer when she was a teenager. But her mother and her sisters never talked about his death after the funeral. "It was like we had to pretend everything was okay. Even when he was really sick and it was clear he was going die, my mother wouldn't discuss it."

"But didn't you and your sisters talk about it?"

"Only in whispers."

One day she came in with her husband. Unbeknownst to me she had decided the three of us would talk about her death.

"So, Bill, Debra's here and I thought we should talk about me dying."

I was surprised, and Bill looked terrified.

"I didn't know, Bill. Honest," I said.

Kari continued. "Well, Bill, I really think you should remarry. Those boys need a mom and you've got to get out and start dating—well, not right away. You know, after maybe a year."

Bill was beet red and his eyes were filled with tears. He sat there silently, swallowing. Kari kept talking in her light and funny way about what to do with her clothes and what to tell the boys, but instead of relaxing Bill, it seemed to paralyze him.

"Bill, breathe," I said. He looked up suddenly as if he forgot I was even in the room.

Kari pressed on. "Promise me you'll speak at my funeral, Debra. You'll be the only one there who can talk about what I really believe."

"I promise."

"But maybe I should go somewhere and not be at home to die. I don't know if the boys should see me wasting away. Debra, what do you think?"

I knew a child's imagination, well, anyone's imagination for that matter, can be worse than the reality. I had been with kids whose parent was taken to the hospital or a hospice facility to die. If they didn't visit frequently, the kids had no idea what was happening. I asked one little boy to draw me a picture of what he thought happened to his mom and he drew this thing that looked like a *meat grinder* with his mom's hands sticking out the top.

I wanted Kari and Bill to understand this, so I told them about Addie Brown, a woman I met with when I worked in hospice.

I had visited Addie in her home for a couple of months. I usually came in the afternoon, and her three grandchildren were always there. After school they came to her house and stayed with her until their mother picked them up after work. This had been going on for years since Addie's daughter was a single mom, and Addie adored her grandkids.

She had lung cancer that had been discovered at a late stage. At the time, it wasn't even treatable with chemotherapy. When it became clear she was too weak to make cookies, or sing and play piano, they put her bed in the living room so she could be "part of the wildness!" as she would say. This way she could still read stories or watch TV with her grandkids. I thought this was great, but her daughter told me this was not a popular decision.

"Her next-door neighbor thinks I'm taking advantage of Mom. She said the children shouldn't see their grandmother like this." She rolled her eyes. "What does 'like this' mean? Mom's getting weaker and thinner, but I think she's even more beautiful."

I had to agree. As Addie's body wasted away, she seemed more spirited than ever. "I am so blessed," she said. "I have these wonderful wild things running around and taking care of me."

Her eldest grandchild, Tess, who was eleven, combed and braided Addie's hair and painted her fingernails sparkly blue. "Looks like I'm already dead," Addie said smiling and surveying her manicure.

"You're right," I said. "Except for the sparkle."

Shauna at eight, was shy and liked to cuddle with Addie, running her plastic ponies up and down the blankets, neighing and snorting, whispering some secret narrative.

Glennie at five was a small tornado. He laid car tracks all over the house, played Nerf baseball in the living room, and pounded on the old upright piano.

"Everyday he climbs up on my bed," Addie told me, "and asks me to tell him a story. And I always do."

Addie was in a coma for about twenty-four hours before she died. The hospice nurse and I arrived soon after. As usual, her grandkids were there, this time they were quietly playing together.

I sat down on the carpet with them. Tess looked up at me. "I brought decals for her nails," she said tearfully. She held out the decals, a set of ten little bumblebees.

"She would have loved them, honey."

Shauna had her horses lying down in a circle. "What's happening with your horses, Shauna?"

"Oh," she said stroking one that had a real mane and tail, "this is what horses do when they're sad."

And then suddenly, as if he couldn't stay still a moment longer, Glennie jumped up.

As he had done every day for months, he climbed up on Addie's bed. "Grandma?" he said softly. Nobody moved or said a word—what if it really was a mistake to let him witness his grandmother's death? Then he climbed right on top Addie's body, straddled her chest and leaned forward. He lifted up her eyelid and looked directly into her eye. "Grandma? Are you in there?"

He paused for a moment and then turned to us with a small grin on his face and said, "She's not in there."

We all smiled back and nodded. And then with the certainty of a five-year-old, he climbed down and said, "Okay." He was perfectly satisfied.

We all breathed a sigh of relief as I had secretly wondered if he was going to be working this out on his shrink's couch for the next forty years. But no, he was not afraid or traumatized.

After I told them about Addie, I could see Kari had completely changed her mind about dying away from home. I turned to Bill and said, "Bill, what do you think?"

"I don't want her shut away," he answered. "But we don't have to think about this anytime soon."

We had to think about it way sooner than anyone liked. Two months later it was clear her disease was progressing, and there was no treatment left for her. And suddenly her willingness to discuss her own death vanished. All she could talk about was the next experimental drug and trying to hang on.

I have seen this before. It's as if once death becomes more of an undeniable reality and less of an abstract concept, the person can no longer speak of it. For some people it is fear and for others I think it is utter disbelief. Kari could not believe she was going to be separated from her children. For her it seemed discussing her death at this point was like agreeing to abandon her boys.

I went to see her in the hospital just before she went home to die. She looked up at me as I walked in. "I hope it doesn't come to this for you."

Up until that moment I had pushed it out of my mind that Kari and I had the same disease. I knew the circumstances were totally different—hers was a later stage, more aggressive, and major lymph node involvement. But with her lying there, her eyes yellow, Bill sitting hunched over the side of her bed, I had to keep reminding myself he was not Wes, and she was not me. My heart was pounding and my stomach curled up into a tight knot. Not Wes. Not me.

"Kari, it's important that you know—" Bill could hardly choke out the words. "You are everything to me. I love you so much."

Her eyes were closed and she squeezed his hand. Not Wes! Not me! Then after a moment she whispered something to him.

"Yes," he said. "Debra, she wants to be sure you will speak, you know—at her funeral."

I was struggling to breath, to swallow, to not break down sobbing. I didn't want her to die. Fuck cancer.

"You promised." She said this in such a loud, strong voice that it startled me. I realized we all had been speaking in whispers.

I managed to swallow down the feather pillow that was stuck in my throat. "Yes, I remember."

"Tell the truth."

"I will."

Then I sat there and held her hand and watched her sleep. My whole body was tense, I swear, every single muscle because I was trying so hard not to cry. Mr. Martha Miyagi? God? Spirit, Universe, Ground of Our Being? Where are you?

In, over, around, and through you.

Then there was a huge Divine sigh. I felt it—soothing, warm, and clean around us like a comforter that has been airing in the sun. Bill felt it, too, because he looked up at me with a slight smile. Swaddled in spirit like newborns. I relaxed in it for a few minutes. Then I kissed her goodbye and left.

Some consider this the hardest part of my job. I consider it the best, the richest, the most sacred. I would never choose not loving my patients to avoid the pain of losing them. That is the risk in loving anybody. But we are never alone with the pain of the loss.

She died two weeks later. Her pastor called me and asked me to choose a Bible verse that reflected my experience with Kari. Picking the scripture was easy because Kari and I had talked about John 15:12. This is where Jesus says to his disciples, "And my command is this, love one another as I have loved you."

I went to the service with her infusion nurse and her case manager. It was on a Saturday, two days post-chemo, which was a bad day for me. I felt tired, nauseous, and headachy. But worst of all, I was wearing an old pair of knee-high nylons (which Wes calls "cheaters") and they were sliding down my calves. I had on a pretty hot-looking, mid-calf, black Liz Claiborne dress, but I was sure these damn cheaters would pool around my ankles like saggy elephant skin.

I walked up to the podium and it took every molecule of self-control not to bend down and pull them up. I took a moment and looked out at the congregation. I could see from their faces they were all kind people. Sitting in the front row with Kari's three little boys was Bill. Okay, so I couldn't look there. I began.

"Whenever patients identify themselves as Christian, I ask them about their faith community. Kari told me about this community and how much she appreciated the love and support she received from all of you. She was so grateful for your phone calls, meals, childcare, rides, and especially your prayers. And I think that truly you loved her as Christ commanded: 'Love one another as I have loved you.'

"Kari was fully engaged in her faith, always questioning her beliefs, wondering about interpretations, and curious about historical context."

I didn't tell them our speculations about the teenage Jesus.

"One of the things I loved about her was she didn't take her faith for granted. She struggled to understand and integrate her beliefs. And she was brave enough to question, reflect on, and even reject some of them."

I didn't say which ones she rejected but I could feel a certain tenseness creep through some of the crowd. Except for her family, that is. Her sisters were looking up at me smiling, and Bill slightly nodded his head.

Kari and I had discussed many verses and agreed if a person could keep the commandment, "Love one another as I have loved you," all the rest would fall into place.

"What exactly does it mean?" she had asked.

"Well, yeah, there's the rub." I had answered. "We spend our entire lives working out what it means to love one another as Christ loved us. A hell of a command."

No doubt about it, it is a command. It's not as if Jesus was making a suggestion like some waiter helping you with your dinner decision, "May I *suggest* loving one another as I have loved you." No, he said, "this is my *command*."

I told the crowd how much Kari loved her family and how hard she had tried to stay alive. Then I told them about the last conversation I had with her.

"After she went into a home hospice program, about a week before she died, I figured it was okay to talk about death again. I said, 'Kari, so now you're pretty clear that you are going to die from this.' And she said, 'I'm doing everything I can, not to. What's the number of your naturopath?'

"If we hadn't talked so openly about death the year before," I said, "I would have been worried. But I knew she was saying this, not because she was afraid of death, but because she loved life so much. She wanted to continue working out the commandment, 'Love one another as I have loved you.'

"Kari died peacefully, surrounded by love. I believe the love of her family and friends helped her let go gently and lightly."

Then I decided to throw in a little Buddhist prayer. "So my prayer today is that in loving one another, we would all be healed, we would all be blessed, and we would all have peace. Amen."

I went back to my seat and pulled up my cheaters. After the service Bill and Kari's sisters embraced me and thanked me.

I kept my promise.

Eight

INFUSED WITH THANKS

Dear Fabulous Friends and Family,

At 7 a.m. on December 8, I quietly, and without ritual, took my last Cytoxan pill. There are a lot of complaints one could make about chemo, but the fact is, it kills cancer cells, and I was grateful for the scientists (and patients) who made it possible. I meditated on that for a few minutes, and then it came to me: if Cytoxan can kill cancer cells, surely it can get rid of that scum in the bottom of my toilet.

I had eight 50-milligram pills left. They were even blue, the traditional color of toilet bowel cleaners. I knew my toilet was eligible for this experiment, so after obtaining informed consent, I carefully dumped the pills in the bowl, and they magically settled on the worse spots. Targeted therapy. When I came back half an hour later, there was a little blue pile of dissolved Cytoxan. Clearly I needed to disperse the drug. I took an old toothbrush (I think it was an old one) and stirred it up. Beautiful aqua blue!

I planned to call my discovery "Cytoiletan." No scrubbing necessary! I could only hope there were no side effects—we've all had the experience of a vomiting toilet, and it's not pretty. I came back in another half hour and flushed. Alas. In spite of my efforts, the aggressive scum continued to grow. My treatment failed the toilet. Procter and Gamble would not be beating down my door. I had to go back to the traditional therapy: Lysol and elbow grease.

In spite of my disappointment that morning, I continued on to the clinic where I spent the day seeing patients. Lots of them. This worked out well for my infusion staff friends who secretly decorated my room for my last treatment. I hadn't a clue.

I walked into what has been variously described as a "Parisian apartment," a "diva salon," or a "high-class bordello." I was immediately presented with a hot pink feather boa and invited to lie on the bed, which was covered with over-sized pillows and a chenille bedspread. There was sparkling cider on ice served in champagne glasses. Windham Hill music was playing, and Christmas lights surrounded a handmade window-sized card. Tablecloths turned the hazardous waste container into an end table. Doilies covered the sharps container. It was no time for a surprise accreditation visit! There were even battery-operated candles! Coffee was served with the lemon tart and white chocolate cake.

I can hardly remember getting my chemo, and when everyone sang the end-of-chemo song, Wes and I both cried. There were all sorts of meaningful things I wanted to say, but my mind was as fuzzy as the chenille bedspread. So let me say them here:

Thank you all for taking care of me. It doesn't matter if you never accessed my port, took a vital sign, brought me a warm blanket, or signed the card. Thanks to anyone who asked me how I was doing, gave me a hug, said hello, sent me an e-mail, a kind thought or a prayer, or took care of me. This is powerful medicine.

I often hear patients say they feel cared for at the SCCA, and I think that is because we are good at simply saying hello, at acknowledging the existence of another person. This is important outside of the clinic, but it really matters inside the clinic because as a patient, it's easy to feel you are a faceless part of the big, sick, cancer crowd. But I think we treat our patients like special individuals, each of us with our own set of symptoms, side effects, and situations. That in itself is healing. So thanks to all of you.

There has been a suggestion from some staff that I keep my port-a-catheter in for demonstration purposes. Just last week we had a patient who had what we call in medical jargon, "really crappy veins." I successfully talked her into getting a port after yanking down my sweater, pointing to my port and saying, "See, it just sits there like a sweet, little gumdrop. And your nurse puts a needle right in the middle of it. You don't have to have your arm mercilessly jabbed, your veins wickedly pricked or a tourniquet torturing your arm." I tried to present this in a neutral, factual way.

In spite of the usefulness of my port, I will get it out at some point soon. But I may use it for an infusion of Zometa because it turns out genetics trump thirty years of running and calcium supplements. I've inherited significant osteoporosis. (See? I'm not as dense as you thought.)

And finally, if you have any housekeeping problems—well, if this tamoxifen doesn't work out you can try "tamoxiclean." I'm sure it will work.

Sincere Thanks, Love, and Hugs,
Debra

Uncharted Territory

When I first met Mike Glazer he was charming to the point of smarmy. He always smiled and raised his eyebrows in the way that says, "I want to have to sex with you."

For example, I'd ask, "Would you like a bottle of water?"

He'd say, "Sure!" and then smile and raise his eyebrows up and down. Ick. He had a perpetual golden-brown tan and wore Hawaiian shirts and flip-flops. Yes, in Seattle. In the winter. He was fifty-six years old and had metastatic rectal cancer.

On my second visit to him, he told two filthy jokes to his infusion nurse and me. I can forgive a dirty joke, but what I can't forgive is an unfunny dirty joke. We wondered if he had a personality change due to steroids, or perhaps a small stroke? Or was he just being a jerk?

I didn't visit him for a few weeks after that. When I saw him again, what he most wanted to talk about was how he wanted a girlfriend and wanted to get laid. He told me his ex-wife thought it was justice he had rectal cancer, because he was such an asshole. It was his affair that broke up their marriage.

"But a man like me has needs," he said. I skillfully steered the conversation away from sex. I felt as if he were testing me, to see if I was put off by all his sexual references. I was mostly bored.

Once we got off sex, he would talk about money: how everything was costing him too much, how he wasn't paid enough at work, how his remarried ex-wife had lots of money. It was tempting to point out that he could save a few bucks by staying off the tanning bed. After a while I wanted to scream at him, "You've got incurable cancer and all you can think about is money?"

So why did I keep visiting him? Because beneath all this Trader Vic, sex god bravado I sensed there was a very frightened man. I also knew his disease was progressing and at some point, facing his death would be undeniable.

In the months that followed I found out he was raised Catholic but rejected Catholicism. He married his wife because he got her pregnant. He divorced when his kids were little, and his wife had custody of them.

"I paid child support," he said. "*That* was a money sucker."

He started coming in for chemo on days I didn't work, so I didn't see him for months. When I finally saw him again, I was almost done with chemo. There was no way I was going to mention that. I'd be crazy to even *think* the word "breast" around him.

He was in Bay 47. I looked in there and then checked the board again. I did not recognize him. He had lost a tremendous amount of weight. Not only that, I was shocked to see how naturally pale he was. He was sitting in his bed, just staring down at his feet. I knocked on the wall before opening the curtain.

"Mike, hi, remember me?"

"Sure, where have you been?"

"Not here the days you were. How are you doing?"

"Not that good." This was the first time he wasn't smiling or raising his eyebrows.

"What's happening?"

"Well, my son is living with me. He takes really good care of me. I'm kinda surprised because I know he's still pissed off at me for leaving his mother. Maybe he's right. Maybe I should have stuck around."

He went on for an hour, talking about his regrets, his sons, his band, and surprisingly, his gratitude for the medical staff. When I asked him about his beliefs around death, all he could say was he wasn't ready to give up. Before I left, for the first time ever, I gave him a hug, and he cried on my shoulder for a few moments. I went right back to my desk to write my chart note.

Chart Note: Spiritual Care

I met with patient in the infusion suite. We have not seen one another for months, so he caught me up on his life. He just bought a house in a Seattle suburb and is looking forward to living there. The stairs in his Downtown condo have become too much for him. He is also grateful to have his eldest son living with him, as he has been an excellent caregiver. There are some unresolved issues between them that can make things stressful for Mike. I suggested this could be an opportunity for them to discuss these things and resolve them.

Mike became quite tearful when talking about the support of his friends. He belongs to an informal band and plays guitar. He feels the band members have really been there for him. He also expressed gratitude for his doctor and for the care he has received at the clinic.

He became tearful when talking about not wanting to "give up." It is difficult for him to discuss his beliefs around death, but we did talk about reframing "giving up" as "letting go."

Mike was raised Catholic but "gave it all up once I moved out of the house." Recently he has made some jokes about sin and Hell and "knowing where I'm going to go." My sense is although he says he has rejected Catholicism, there are still some beliefs he holds. At this point he is unable to articulate his spiritual beliefs.

We discussed how he is "having a hard time looking in the mirror." Mike has lost over fifty pounds and looks quite different from when I saw him last. Although thin, I let him know I found him to be very "Clint Eastwood-y" in his gauntness. I assured him this was not a bad look for him, although perhaps he should try to gain a bit more weight—or start wearing a cowboy hat.

I will continue to offer spiritual and emotional support.

Years ago there was a chaplain in the department who was known for her brief chart notes. She would often write something like, "I visited the patient in his room. Then I left." She felt it was nobody's business what went on between the chaplain and a patient.

I had a slightly different view. I wrote chart notes for many reasons. Chaplains have a pretty low profile, and I think having a chart note is a good way to let the staff know we exist. Reading our notes gives them some idea of what we do. Of course, I don't usually put in details about recipe swapping or a patient's feeling about the Mariners' pitching. I try to make my notes relevant and at least interesting.

I never knew who would be reading my note. We are always warned, "Don't write anything you wouldn't want read aloud in a court of law." That was probably the wrong thing to tell me, because I imagined some well-dressed lawyer reading my note aloud and the judge saying, "What an insightful, provocative note. I must retire to my chambers to think it about it."

I also wrote notes on what I thought was important for the health care team to know. In Mike's case I thought they should know we had a conversation about dying, that death was on his radar screen. Perhaps this would make it easier for his physician to talk about chemo failing and when to stop. The note would also give her a clue that it was difficult for him to talk about death, but at least the subject had been broached.

Maybe she would pick up on the fact there was some unfinished business between him and his son, and that might influence her decision around stopping treatment. Noting he was tearful and he was grateful for his friends was a message he wasn't the macho jerk that he seemed to be. I also wanted her to know in spite of the fact he was usually arrogant and demanding, he was grateful for his doctor's care. And anyone who knew Mike Glazer and read my remark about him looking "Clint Eastwood-y" would understand immediately how important that was to him.

Another reason I wrote notes was purely for myself because I couldn't remember a damn thing. Once I read my note, it all came back to me. I think the reason I can't remember all my patients and our conversations is it isn't healthy to keep all those people in my head. This happens to the nurses, too. We all agree there are some patients, who are unforgettable, but 90 percent of them go out of our brains and it's probably better that way.

The last reason I chart is more subversive: I didn't think it was a bad idea for the reader to ponder the very thing a patient and I had been pondering, that is, what happens when you die? What has my life meant? What is it like for me to look in the mirror these days? So a chart note could *secretly* be like a little homily or meditation. Subliminal spiritual direction.

Most patients don't even realize both chaplains and social workers chart at all. One patient was very upset with her social worker and said she felt betrayed, as if she told a girlfriend a secret who then told everyone. For a while that caused many of us to write the vaguest and most useless notes. It's true patients have the right to read their charts, so it's a fine line we tread.

As a rule, I don't chart gory details. For example, if a patient and I talk about her being abused as a child, I write, "discussed painful childhood issues."

Sometimes I walk out of a patient's room and wonder, what just happened? Charting is a good way of sorting that out. It is also a way of cleansing myself, of letting one patient go, so I can be present for the next one.

"I will continue to follow and offer spiritual and emotional support." I almost always write that at the end of every note unless I'm not planning on seeing the patient again. I never write "give" emotional and spiritual support, but "offer" it. You can't give support unless it's accepted, so all you can promise to do is offer it.

Last Pill and Testament

Even on days I wasn't getting chemo, I was offered, and gratefully accepted lots of support from the staff. I received holy oil from Jerusalem, rosary beads from the Vatican, and impromptu shoulder rubs. On chemo days the nurses often gave Wes and me leftover box lunches to take home for dinner. This was such a godsend. On those dark winter nights after chemo, shopping for groceries felt like going out into the forest to kill a stag for dinner.

Early on people had asked, "Who will be a chaplain to the chaplain?" The answer turned out to be: everybody. I didn't have deep, soul-baring conversations with everyone, but it seemed everyone was *willing*. Not a day went by when someone didn't ask me, "How are you feeling?" and then left room, left space for my answer. And I could answer big or I could answer small. But there was always space for the big answer. Just as importantly, nobody pressed me with, "Really—how *are* you?" when I wanted to give a small answer.

I was so very happy to be done with chemo. It meant the end to constant low-grade nausea, the return of my taste buds and my energy, and the freedom to be away for more than six days. I was also grateful my colleagues no longer had to deal with caring for one of their own. As much as I tried to let go of this, it weighed heavily upon me. I knew as time went on, it became *easier* for the staff to treat me, but it was never *easy*.

But it's tricky business deciding how to proceed after finishing chemo. It's tempting to think, "Now I can go back to my life." But as they say, you can never go back, you simply redefine what is normal—the "new normal."

For all cancer survivors, there is always a chance of recurrence, even if it's only a teeny, tiny, quark-sized chance. Knowing this makes some people afraid to celebrate. They feel as if they are tempting fate.

Joyce was a perfect example of this. She was from Alaska and had been diagnosed with an early stage breast cancer and received the same chemotherapy I did.

"We threw a big party," she said. "I thought we were done with it and I could go back to my life." A year later she had a recurrence, and a year after that metastases to her bones and her brain. "I thought I had beat cancer. But now I wish I hadn't celebrated. I wish I had been more respectful of it."

I didn't want to treat cancer like a god, an entity to whom I had to show respect. I didn't think of cancer as Arnold Schwarzenegger in *The Terminator* saying, "I'll be back." I felt more like Dorothy in *The Wizard of Oz*. I had escaped the wicked witch of the West and her flying monkeys. I was back in Kansas, and I wanted to celebrate and say thanks. If it recurs, it recurs. Why miss a party now for something that may or may not happen?

There is another tricky part of finishing chemo, and because I worked at the clinic, it was one I didn't have to contend with: leaving my caregivers and the safety of the medical community.

Yes, people are thrilled to be out of the weekly chemo rut, but after seeing the infusion staff weekly for six months or more, they form a close bond with them that makes it hard to leave. Many patients cry at their last chemotherapy, tears of happiness at finishing, but also tears of sadness.

One patient told me it was like cutting an umbilical cord. "There is always someone to call about any little symptom or problem. Now I feel like I'm out there on my own, and what if I get a headache or a fever? I guess I do what a regular person would do—take aspirin." As much as you want your normal life back, it's kind of cool to have a benevolent "mom" taking your temperature, your pulse, and fussing about your health every week.

Often patients want to stay connected to their care providers, but some staff members have very clear boundaries and don't keep in touch with patients once they are outside the system. Others are more relaxed about it.

I don't have boundaries exactly—more of a selectively permeable membrane, which allows some people to stay in, and not others. There are patients I never see again, those with whom I keep in e-mail contact, others who have been to my home for dinner and stayed overnight, and one who has become a mentor and close friend to me.

Rock Music

When a patient has his or her last treatment, we gather round, sing the end-of-chemo song, blow bubbles, and bestow a plastic crown and lei. Then we take their photo. But sometimes we also do the rock ritual.

We do this for patients with whom we feel very close or who live in another state, or who we feel need to take something tangible with them to remind them of our support. We did it for Jenny because she was only in her twenties and lived on one of the islands off the coast. Jenny's mother died of cancer when she was a child.

Her nurses and I gathered around her bed. "Jenny," I said, "each of us has different strengths that have helped us get through tough times. So each of us will put our strength in this rock for you to call on any time you need it."

Her chemo nurse started. "Jenny, I put into this rock my ability to see the big picture. This has kept me from getting down about the little things and lets me know there is more to life than just me and my problems."

"I put patience into this rock," her case manager said. "I know you will need a pretty big dose of patience as your health and your hair slowly return."

I went last. "Jenny, I put into this rock my sense of humor. It has saved me from taking myself too seriously." Of course I wanted to say something really funny to *prove* I had a sense of humor, but nothing came. At this point tears were streaming down Jennifer's face. We always finish the ritual with me playing my cedar flute.

I am not some big virtuoso on this flute. I used to play my recorder for my hospice patients, but this turned out to be a failure for several reasons. One was I would get too worked up about playing the wrong notes or the wrong rhythm. The other was a soprano recorder can be a little shrill, especially in the hands of an amateur, and not at all soothing to patients.

One day I was at an Earth Day fair out on Bainbridge Island. A man was standing in front of a table with dozens of wooden flutes on it. I picked up a small cedar one. The guy behind the counter said, "Just keep your ring finger down and you can play anything." I played a few notes on it, and I loved it. It was nothing like my recorder. It had a soft, haunting sound.

"I'll take it," I said.

"Oh, wonderful. Then you'll want to know it's a pentatonic scale and—"

I cut him off. "No. I don't want to know anything about it."

He paused, looked at me and said, "Oh, I see—you want to play from your heart."

"Yes, that's right." And that is what I did. I never worried about hitting the wrong notes because there were no wrong notes. I was perfectly relaxed, because I made it up as I went along. Mindful of the use of cedar in prayer, before I played I always took a good long sniff of my flute—to remind me my music was a prayer.

A Bride in Me

On Wes and my tenth anniversary we had a huge party and invited all our guests to come dressed in their wedding clothes. That's right, they wore the clothes in which they were married. (Well, okay, there were ten women in their actual wedding gowns. About half the women didn't own them anymore, and everybody else couldn't fit into them. The men got off easy since tuxedo trousers have those expandable waistbands.)

We moved all of the furniture out of the living room and hired a little three-piece combo. I made fabulous finger food and a three-tiered wedding cake with our original ornament. Even though she had never married, I made a wedding gown with a tulle train for our dog, Cokey. It featured a silk poinsettia, beading, and two-inch lace. She also wore pearls.

I was definitely channeling Martha Stewart. I made tiny bouquets for the brides to throw, and tiny garters for the men to fling. We gave small "wedding" gifts to all our guests, since they were, after all, brides and grooms.

To say it was hilarious is an understatement. When would you ever see so many brides at one reception? There were wedding gowns there from the 1960s to the 1990s. In short, we ate, we drank, we danced. It had been the best party we'd ever given, and people called the next day begging us to do it again. We had promised we'd do it in ten years.

So here it was ten years later, our twentieth anniversary—and the day before my last chemo. There was no way we were having a big party. I could barely stay up until 8 p.m. every night. So I said to Wes, "Well, let's just you and I go out for dinner and wear our wedding clothes." He agreed because he is a really good sport about stuff like this.

Our anniversary was on a weeknight, so I brought my gown to the clinic. The nurses were enthusiastic about this. At 5 p.m. two of them helped me get dressed while another took pictures. It was just like having bridesmaids, except they were all wearing lab coats and stethoscopes. Then they made me walk down the hall past all the patient rooms because there is something really fun and exciting and slightly crazy about seeing a bride in a cancer center.

My dress was not a simple, modern column dress. It had an enormous skirt, big puffy lace sleeves, and a train; all of which add up to miles of fabric. It made a lot of noise when I walked because I was wearing a big stiff crinoline slip underneath. The patients started popping out of their rooms like prairie dogs.

"Are you getting married?" one man asked me.

"No, just going out to dinner," I answered.

My promenade down the hall delighted everyone. Patients and staff alike were smiling like crazy. What's not to like about a bride? It's the same way when someone brings a baby into the clinic. I don't know how it is for an infant, but I was thrilled to provide enjoyment just by walking around. Today was my anniversary, tomorrow was my last chemo. I was bursting with joy.

Wes and I agree to meet at this fancy little French restaurant called Rover's. It's the kind of place you go to celebrate and the owner comes out wearing his famous hat and schmoozes with you. Most importantly, we heard the food was excellent.

The nurses help me bustle up the train, but when I got into my car, it came unhooked. I stuffed the train onto the passenger seat. It looked like the air bag had gone off. The train kept falling off the seat onto my filthy floor mat. I reached over, grabbed the seatbelt, brought it across the train and belted it in. Now I had a stiff white mummy leaning against the window.

The parking lot was up the street, a block from the restaurant. Even though it was only 5:30 p.m., it was already pitch dark and cold. But I wasn't cold, because I was conveniently having a hot flash. Besides, what kind of coat could I wear over this enormous dress? So I walked down Madison Street, carrying my train over one arm, car keys in hand. The same thing that happened in the clinic happened on the street. People came out of stores smiling like crazy. Other people on the street stopped dead in their tracks.

"Hey, hello there—bride!"

"Merry Christmas!"

"Oh, my goodness, look at that dress!"

Two people were smiling but speechless, and came up to shake my hand. It was as if I were giving off some kind of fumes that made everyone euphoric. I suddenly realized I could bring joy to the world by simply walking down the street at night in my wedding dress. I felt high myself, as high as I felt twenty years ago walking down the aisle and out of the church with my new husband.

I arrived at the restaurant about ten minutes before they opened, so I stood out on their little porch. I could see someone looking out at me, and then the door opened and the mâitre d' said, "Madam, would you like to come in?"

"Yes! We have reservations."

"I thought so."

He found our names and then asked, "Is there anything I can do for you while you wait?"

"Well, yes. Do you know how to bustle a train?"

"No—but it's always a good time to learn."

We picked through the mountain of fabric and lace and found the two hooks on the train that fastened to my dress. Then I stood happily waiting in the lobby.

In the meantime, Wes was getting dressed at Harborview, the county hospital. He came out of the men's room in his tux. The janitor, pushing his cart down the hall, stopped and looked at him.

"Nice duds, dude."

He snagged a ride with another physician who lived in the area and arrived about five minutes after me. They sat us at a table that was smack in the middle of the room and gave us two glasses of champagne. I loved it even though it tasted like gasoline to me.

We ordered, and then Wes got up. I couldn't help thinking, "Holy Cow, we just got here and you have to pee already? Maybe you should get your prostate checked." But he didn't leave; he got down on one knee.

Before I tell you what happened next, you should know that when Wes proposed to me, I was sitting on the living room couch in his San Francisco condo reading the morning paper. He was in the kitchen making coffee and yelled out, "Hey, you know what?"

"What?" I yelled back.

"Well, I was thinking—I've analyzed things and what you want to do with your life is compatible with what I want to do with my life. So I think getting married would work."

"Okay. That would be a blast!" Then he finished making coffee. We weren't even in the same room.

So there we were at Rover's and he was down on one knee and said, "I think I didn't do it properly before. I love you, Debra, will you marry me?"

Then he reached into his pocket and snapped open this ring box that had a gorgeous diamond ring in it. He put it on my finger, and of course I start weeping. Wes tried to get up gracefully, but he's got a bad knee and lost his balance and grabbed the table to steady himself. The table started to fall, but I took hold of it with both hands so tears were streaming unchecked down my face when the waiter arrived with little complimentary hors d'oeuvres and said, "Oh, my."

Wes made it back into his seat, and by then I was outright crying, I stuck out my hand and said to the waiter, "Ooh, heja gayma dimoning."

He set the plates down, smiled, and said, "Stunning." I realized we were going to have to leave him a big tip.

I sat there looking at this dazzling ring and staring at my husband who was the most beautiful man I knew. What if I hadn't met Wes? I was astonished I could be falling in love with my husband all over again. I was overwhelmed by gratitude and my whole body tingled as if a current was running through it. I felt the Presence vibrating in every cell of my body. We sat there holding hands across the table, very still, not needing to speak. Then the waiter brought my bottle of water and broke the spell.

One of the wonderful things about this restaurant is that the dining is leisurely, say, three hours for a five-course meal. This is terrific if you don't go to bed at 8:00 p.m. I felt my energy draining away, like sand in an hourglass. The chef came out and schmoozed with us. We told him we loved the food, although at that point I could have gone facedown into the pâté. We declined dessert. Wes would have had to feed it to me after strapping me into the chair.

Rover's was the kind of place where no one was crass enough to just walk up to your table and say, "So did you two just get married or something?" No, no, they were very discreet—they asked the waiter.

So when we got up to leave, everyone clapped and said, "Congratulations!"

I cried all the way out to the car.

Sighed Effects

The list of side effects from chemo is long and includes common ones such as nausea, headache, fatigue, hair thinning, hot flashes, insomnia, constipation—well, let's just stop there. They told me about most of them, but there were some side effects no one mentioned. These included: a new appreciation for my friends, a deep tenderness between Wes and me, and finding numerous wave-lengths through which I was hearing the Spirit.

My friends were fabulous about bringing food and cards and flowers. But what astonished me was how I felt their prayers. Sometimes in the middle of the night I would lie there, wide-awake, and a warm sparkly feeling of being held, of being loved, would come over me. The next day someone would say to me, "I was praying for you last night when I got up to pee."

The Powerful Pee Prayer. Why isn't this in any books on spiri-tuality or mysticism? That middle-of-the-night appeal whispered between getting out of, and getting back into bed. A prayer said while performing a humble bodily function; the opposite end of the spectrum from having an entire High Mass said for you.

Don't you think Jesus just loves this? That is so totally up his alley, right up there with the manger and the lowing cattle. Ordi-nary. Simple. Powerful.

I knew cancer could bring a couple closer, but I had also seen it tear a couple apart.

Wes and I became closer in a way that comes from being utterly vulnerable with one another. It wasn't that we hadn't talked about dying before. Wes had always been convinced he would die first, and he would go *on* about how I should date and where the life insurance policy was. But now he wasn't so sure who was going to die first, and that was a good thing.

We became intensely aware of life's unpredictability, which made us say, "God willing," after, "I'll be home around seven." We never left without kissing one another, even if one of us was leaving the house at 5 a.m. We never hung up without saying, "I love you."

I'm sure it made people just want to throw up when we kissed in a restaurant before one of us got up to use the bathroom. But you never know what can happen on the way to the toilet! Sud-den stroke. Drive-by shooting. Alien abduction.

We felt a deep tenderness for one another that caused us to be even kinder to each other. Both of us let things go, didn't have to be right, and didn't insist on our way. The kinder he was to me, the kinder I was to him, and it simply grew.

Well, all right—I was still a Nazi in the kitchen, a bossy, snippy know-it-all. A kitchen bully.

Then again, in spite of my having *cancer*, Wes *still* doesn't squeeze out the kitchen sponge. Or fill the pepper shakers—which I never use. But I let the clothes wrinkle in the dryer. So we haven't exactly perfected things.

Besides the cedar tree in the fence, I heard the Spirit speak to me in lots of new ways. The most amazing was out of my own mouth. Athletes talk about being in "the zone," a place where every action seems perfect and effortless. Chaplains, too, can get in the zone. I would be talking to a patient and thoughts and ideas I didn't even know I *had* started coming out of my mouth. The patient would be nodding and saying something like, "Yes, exactly. So true. I see what you mean."

On the surface it sounded as if I was offering some spiritual insight. But here's the irony: the words were meant for me!

So I'm listening to a patient tell me how she has such guilt about not doing enough, there's housework and exercise and a book club and gardening. There's always so much to do and so much guilt about not being productive. Where did that guilt come from and how could she find time to meditate?

I said, "Yeah, I'm curious where it comes from, but I guess what's important is to get off the Activity Train. You go whooshing through life, never stopping and enjoying where you are, because you are nowhere really—just racing. Maybe that's what meditation is about: stepping off the train and exploring your inner space."

The whole time I was speaking this woman was nodding her head and saying, "Absolutely. Yes, you're right."

There wasn't even a nanosecond for me to be pleased with myself, because I knew instantly the words were meant for me. I couldn't stand being such a fraud, so I said, "Of course, I am speaking to myself, as well."

The Peanut Is Brittle

I couldn't wait for my DEXA bone density scan. This was one area where I knew I'd be strong. Thirty years of running and all those damn calcium pills on which I nearly choked to death every day. Well, it was worth it because it would serve me now.

I absolutely swaggered into radiology feeling this was a test for which I had been studying. This was an exam I would ace.

So, of course, I just about fell over when my report came back telling me not only did I have osteopenia, a decrease in bone density, but significant osteoporosis, which is considered a *disease.*

"High risk for hip fracture," the report said. Impossible! I actually called radiology and asked if they mixed up my report with someone else's—with some elderly person who didn't exercise and take her calcium.

I said before that cancer messes with your self-image. Mine required some adjustment as I chose to see my white cells as "sensitive," as opposed to "wimpy." This diagnosis of osteoporosis was more shocking to me than my cancer diagnosis. I had always thought of myself as having strong bones like a mighty Alaskan bear. Now they were telling me I had the bones of a hummingbird.

It reminded me once again how little control I really had. So this scan was in fact a test, a test of how flexible I could be, of how quickly I could accept this news and get on with life. Would I be able to keep my equanimity?

I didn't have time to dwell on any of this because I was to meet Beth and her husband Charlie in the clinic sanctuary. She had completed treatment, was moving back to Montana, and she wanted me to teach them how to pray—together.

The first time I ever got a request to give prayer instruction, I stuttered and said something about having an ongoing commentary with the Divine and how maybe I wasn't the best person to instruct them in prayer. I felt both Mr. Martha Miyagi and Jesus just rolling their divine eyes.

You're a minister for Christ's sake. It's part of your job description.

Yeah, for my sake!

Jesus always likes to chime in.

Beth and Charlie had both been raised in conservative Christian churches, but their spiritual beliefs were now far from conservative. What could I teach them that they could do together and was slightly familiar and yet different?

I asked them to sit with their feet flat on the floor, with their hands resting upon one another in their laps "like the Buddha." They had explored enough religions to know what that meant.

"So for five minutes just sit and watch your breath," I said. "No need to change it in any way. Simply focus on your breath and if your attention wanders, which it will, gently bring it back to your breath."

"What should I be saying?" Charlie asked.

"Nothing," I answered. "Just watch your breath. After five minutes I'll say 'palms down' and you can place your hands on your thighs palms down, because you will be releasing anything you want: fears, thoughts, desires, thanks, whatever. After three minutes I'll say, 'palms up' so you are in a posture of receiving from God. Maybe you'll receive an insight now, or maybe it will come later."

"How long is this going to take?" Charlie asked.

"Five plus three plus three equals eleven minutes, which is about the amount of time you spend watching commercials in a half hour television show."

"Hmph," he said. Beth winked at me.

And so we sat, hands like the Buddha, breathing. My mind was a hyperactive marching band consisting mainly of tubas and trumpets with the bass drum banging loudly on one syllable. The band played only one song that went like this: "OsteopoROsis! OsteopoROsis!" Then the piccolos came in with: "OsteoPEEEEEnia! OsteoPEEEEEnia!"

After five minutes I said, "Palms down."

I could still hear the band in the distance. Palms down. Letting go of having things the way I want them. Palms down. Letting go of my expectations. Palms down. Release my perception of what it means to be strong.

I opened one eye and checked my watch. "Palms up," I whispered. The minute you do this, you feel like a child trick-or-treating on Halloween: open, eager, curious, expectant. It's not so much, "*Will* you give to me?" but "*What* will you give to me?"

Despite the fact that talking people and laundry carts constantly go by the sanctuary, I heard nothing but a calm, bright silence. In my mind I saw snow falling softly at night past the moon, past the stars. Everywhere I looked snow was falling on rocks and hills and trees. Beautiful sparkling flakes, a multitude of snowflakes, like blessings piling up around me.

I was raised in the San Francisco Bay Area. It doesn't usually snow there. It doesn't snow that often in Seattle. So I can't tell you why my mind turned into a mystical snow globe. But I can tell you that it was perfect, untroubled happiness.

I don't know how much time passed, but I gradually came to a sense of myself and very quietly said, "Allow your hands to rest upon one another again. And when you're ready, open your eyes."

I could tell Charlie didn't want to come back. Beth slowly opened her eyes and looked at the ground. Finally Charlie opened his, stared at his shoes for a moment, and then looked up at me.

"This is something we can do together at home," he noted quietly.

"Yes." I don't know why we were speaking in whispers, only that it seemed like the thing to do. I think this is probably how the Wise Men were talking around the baby Jesus in the manger. I just can't see them slapping one another on the back and yelling, "Yee-haw! It's the Messiah!"

We sat quietly for a few moments. I felt as if we just woke up from a communal dream, but I didn't ask them about it. It felt too much like asking, "Was it good for you?" There are some things that are best left unexpressed. Yes, this is coming from me, Miss Tell Me Everything. They thanked me and we hugged goodbye.

That night in bed I read this from the Sufi mystic Rumi: "All day I think about it, then at night I say it. Where did I come from, and what am I supposed to be doing? My soul is from elsewhere, I'm sure of that, and I intend to end up there."

I felt I was doing exactly what I was supposed to be doing. But was it possible that my soul was from a place of gently falling snow?

Nine

FLASH IN THE PAN

Dear Fabulous Friends and Family,

It's been a wonderful couple of months of drinking wine and eating chocolate. I no longer have to think about wearing port-accessible clothes. Saliva has returned from its pilgrimage to Spit Mecca and once again resides in my mouth.

You may remember I said I would share any gold nuggets I am able to mine from this experience. There are days when I feel as if I have a glimmer of understanding about life. There are also days when I am awed by how little I understand. And then there are days where I am just odd.

For example, last month Wes had a science meeting in Carmel. We were renting a car to drive from San Jose to Carmel. The nice lady at the rental car agency tried to talk us into an upgrade.

"You know for thirty dollars a day more, I can get you into one of our prestige cars. A Lexus, or perhaps a Jaguar."

"We want the economy car."

"If you join our Gold Member Club today, I can waive the fee for the prestige car."

"We want the economy car."

"There's a Jaguar sitting right out there. For just thirty dollars a day more—"

At that moment I felt because we had to listen to her little schpiel, she could just listen to mine.

"If gas were fifty cents a gallon, we might think about it. I'm a minister—what do I want with a Jaguar?" (Let me point out I never took a vow of poverty.)

She sniffed. "Sometimes it's just a matter of comfort."

I should never have told her I was a minister. I don't often trot out that little fact, but since I had, I guess I thought I should give her a full-blown sermon.

"You know, the Buddhists say it is not a good thing to get addicted to comfort. In fact, that's my resolution for this year—to be comfortable with discomfort."

We finally got the keys to a Ford Focus that had a broken seat, broken armrest, and a trunk that you couldn't open. But hey! I was comfortable with discomfort! Until the *nuclear hot flashes*.

There I was at the science meeting cocktail party wearing nice, warm, corduroy pants, a sweater, a leather jacket, and a backpack purse. I was holding a plate of hors d'oeuvres in one hand, a glass of wine in the other, when suddenly the very center of my head became a pile of hot coals, and my own flesh began to cook from the inside out. Got to get out of the jacket! I looked desperately around for a place to set down my plate. No tables—just groups of happy, cool people.

"So you're from the University of Washington?" a woman asked.

"No, my husband is. I'm not in science. I'm—cooking," I said blinking sweat out of my eye.

"Cooking. Do you own a restaurant?"

"No, I—" The sweater was one of those hairy Angora things. I felt as if I were in the Mojave Desert wearing a leather jacket filled with evil guinea pigs. Have to get outside! Okay, my name is Debra Jarvis, and I'm addicted to comfort. The Buddhists are out of their no-minds!

"Please—excuse me." I ran out the door, set down my food and drink on the nearest bench, and tore off my jacket. I dug through my purse for my fan and then collapsed on a stone wall fanning myself and mopping my face with my cocktail napkin.

"It gets pretty hot when there are so many people in there."

I was shocked to realize there was a man sitting on the other end of the wall. I knew he was a scientist from his name badge.

I explained chemo had fried my ovaries sunny-side-up, and so now I was in abrupt menopause. He clucked sympathetically.

Then he said, "I'm a cancer survivor, too."

He told me several years ago he was diagnosed with lymphoma, and had gone to the Dana-Farber Cancer Institute in Boston to get a bone marrow transplant. They were waiting to get some new protocol up and running, so they delayed his transplant. He was worried about the delay. But while he was waiting for his transplant, he had a spontaneous remission.

"Wow!" I said. "What do you make of that?"

"Well, of course, there's an explanation. My blood made some tumor killing cells."

"But what about the fact that your transplant was delayed?"

He was silent for so long that I finally said, "I bet as a scientist it's hard to accept the mystery of that."

"Yes, it is. But I do."

If he hadn't had to wait, his body would not have had time to heal itself. What he was most worried about, the delay, is what allowed his healing. His story reminded me that often the healing, the miracle, happens while we're waiting or when we're looking the other way. Then—like a cat that has crept silently into the room—we suddenly find the miracle in our laps.

"By the way," I said, "what's your area of research?"

"Cancer," he answered.

He was a scientist, a person who looks for explanations and understanding, yet even he recognized a mystery. Perhaps it's what we do with our mysteries that is most important. He decided to study his.

The dreaded hot flash led me to this man and his miracle story. I think this mystery is one to be shared, not studied.

Love and Hugs,
Debra

Growth Spurt

You can never predict if or when people will grow from their cancer experience. Cece was the perfect example. She was a jet-setting clothing designer and flew all over the world and wore great clothes and shoes. Then she was diagnosed with breast cancer. I met her the day she came in for her first infusion. I walked in her room, and I could feel the anger radiating out of her. It was like standing next to a bonfire. She took one look at me, and I could tell she was furious. In spite of this I visited her during her six months of chemotherapy.

We kept in touch, and a year later we went out for lunch.

"There's something I've been meaning to say to you," she began.

How can you not get nervous when somebody says that? It's like when someone starts out, "No offense—"; nothing good can ever come after that. But I forced myself to smile at Cece and say, "What's that?"

"When I first met you, well, I was so angry and bitter that you were beautiful and healthy. I felt all the healthy people were looking at me with pity. I was enraged every time I came in for chemo. But you never flinched."

"Oh, I flinched," I said. "You just didn't see me."

"Yes, but you kept coming back."

"I knew you would work through it."

"That's nice of you to put it that way," she said. "But I felt more like a kid kicking and screaming and having a tantrum. I can't believe I finally found some inner peace."

"How do you explain it?" I asked because I'm always on the lookout for ways to find inner peace.

"Well, I was sort of forced to lie still for a few months. It was only after I got quiet that I could hear God. I thought I was a good enough person and didn't really need God. I never thought too deeply about anything, but boy, does having cancer make you think. And I found that all the superficial crap I worried about working in the fashion industry is just that—crap. It's really fun when you are twenty but sad when you are forty and still worrying about what other people think of you."

It's pretty common to have a time lag between diagnosis and treatment and spiritual growth. Patients have said to me, "I'm trying to grow from this, I'm trying to find meaning, but I just can't stop crying."

I usually say, "Maybe it's too soon to grow, and all you can do is feel shitty right now." I know what it's like to be a pain-avoiding overachiever, and I learned you couldn't rush personal and spiritual growth. If you could, I would have done it all in high school while I was dealing with acne and feeling overweight. But you can't and there is an undeniable incubation period between trauma and growth.

That's why I love seeing patients a few years after they've completed treatment. They've come out of the mine and have had time to sort through the bag of rocks and pick out the gold nuggets. They've crossed the rope bridge, have made it to the other side, and can look over what they've just crossed and discover who they have become.

The Days of Wine and Chocolate

I'm not a big drinker. What I really missed about not be able to drink wine was the ritual. I missed the way Wes would ask, "Shall we open some wine?" as we were rooting through the refrigerator getting dinner together.

I would laugh when he opened the bottle with that silly, rabbit-shaped opener, because every time he would say proudly,

"So easy!" I loved the sound and smell of the wine being poured, the clink of the glasses, the kiss. We tried to keep the ritual with Crystal Light, but it wasn't the same.

It reminded me of youth pastors who, in trying to be hip, used Coke and M&Ms for Communion. *Please.* I suppose if you were trapped in a snack shack at the county fair and that's all there was, and you wanted to receive Communion because it was clear you were going to die before someone rescued you, well, *then* I think it's okay.

Anyway, at first when wine started tasting bad to me Wes would say, "Let's open a different bottle! Maybe this one is too dry." But when we had so many open bottles that it looked like a wine tasting, he realized it was useless. After a while he stopped drinking wine, too.

I think everyone with cancer struggles to keep domestic rituals. Nancy finished six months of chemotherapy and had a mastectomy. Her three-year-old son Riley was used to snuggling up to her every night before bed.

"So we told him Mommy has a "soft" side and a "tender" side, and he could snuggle only on the soft side."

"Was he able to remember that?" I asked.

"Oh, yeah," she answered. "I started to shake hands with my doctor and Riley piped up, 'That's her tender side!'"

You just do what you can to keep life normal. The hardest ritual for me to keep was eating dinner with Wes. About halfway through my chemo was when everything changed. It was as if my taste buds, who all these years had been wearing khakis and polo shirts, suddenly started wearing leather vests and jackboots.

To me, eating was more than simply putting food in your mouth, chewing, and then swallowing. I could do that. But what I couldn't do was enjoy the same foods he did. All I wanted to

eat was pineapple, pickles, nopalitos, sour olives, and salad with
Italian dressing.

So gone were the moments when we would take a bite of
something, look at each other and say, "M-m-m-m-m." Eating was
no longer a shared experience.

The only exception to this was steak. I was anemic, and my
oncologist was pushing red meat like a waiter with last night's special. I was thrilled we could eat steak together, and I was thrilled
we could afford it. But Wes comes from a happy family of heart
disease, so we really didn't do it too often.

I said, "If you have a heart attack and die because we've been
eating steak because I had cancer—" Well, I couldn't even finish
that sentence. It was too ridiculous.

So I was looking forward to being able to eat again. I somehow
thought I would wake up one morning and, *ta-da*, the taste buds
would be back! But that's not how it happened. It was gradual like
an incoming tide. About two weeks after my last chemo, I found
myself eating a piece of cheddar cheese that had formerly tasted
like Playdough. A few days after that I sipped some wine—not
exactly drinkable, but getting there.

At Christmas a friend arrived at my door carrying an elaborate
two-foot-tall chocolate Santa Claus. His eyebrows and beard were
in white chocolate. His belt buckle and boot were in dark chocolate. I was stunned at his size.

"All I can tell you," she said, "is it didn't look this big in the
catalogue." Everyone who came over took a picture with the giant
chocolate Santa.

I didn't want to cut into the Santa until I was sure chocolate
tasted good to me again. This was no drugstore chocolate Santa, it
was Dilettante chocolate. I wanted the day to be something special. And it was—the Academy Awards.

I wish I could tell you I did this delicately, like some kind of skilled surgeon. But the truth is, somewhere between Best Animated Short Film and Achievement in Costume Design, I took a cleaver and whacked off his head. His head broke into several pieces, the largest of which was his face. I dumped it into a little bowl.

"Eeww," said Wes. "I don't think I can eat him with his face looking up at me."

"Okay, I'll take care of it." I took one last look into Santa's chocolate brown eyes and carefully placed his face into my mouth. He was delicious—just like I remembered chocolate. That was my defining moment, that's how I knew I was getting something resembling my old life back.

But I know it's different for everyone.

"I think what I loved most was getting my fingernails back," Mary told me. She grew up in Britain and always wore suits to her infusions. Her fingernails were a mess from the Adriamycin, so she began wearing gloves to the clinic. The first time she did this, I made her a cup of tea in one of our paper cups and brought it to her on a plastic tray.

"Your tea, madam." She loved it and it became our little ritual to have tea together.

"Yes, most definitely, I loved having nails again because it had been so painful to handle things, to type, to dial the telephone. But sadly my allergies came back once the effects of chemotherapy receded. And my family became less respectful of me and began to argue and behave poorly again. They actually told me they didn't want to hear any more about my cancer."

"Families—you gotta love 'em," I said facetiously.

"On the contrary. My wellness has meant that I make choices toward my friends and away from my immediate family because I simply will *not* tolerate bad treatment any longer. Cancer has taught me it's quite all right to avoid predictably stressful situations. I spent Thanksgiving with friends instead of family."

A lymphoma patient, who was an infectious disease doctor, told me he was obsessed with a fear of infection. So he didn't ride public transit, and even though swimming was his favorite activity, he wouldn't go in a swimming pool.

"I knew I survived," he said, "when I got back in the pool and cranked out my first half-mile. I hadn't been in the pool for over a year, and that first swim was my equivalent of crossing the English Channel."

Lots of people talk about being able to drink wine again, eat spicy food without reflux, play with their kids, walk up a hill without getting out of breath, go all day without a nap, and read serious literature, not just magazines. Things are getting back to normal when people ask, "How are you?" as a passing remark. For many women the sign things were on the upswing came through initiating sex.

"I knew I was better when I was the one to say, 'Hey, I'm interested,'" Sarah said. "Trust me, this was a change from life during six months of chemo! We were on the phone with each other, and my husband was so surprised he rushed home, went running around the house, and had all of his clothes off by the time he ran into the bedroom! It was fantastic! I felt sexy and alive! This was about three weeks after my mastectomy."

But for some people it takes longer to feel they have their lives back. Marie was eight months out of chemo, and had bi-lateral mastectomies and radiation when I talked with her.

"I don't feel like I do have my life back," she said. "But I went out for dinner recently and was in the bathroom applying lip gloss when a woman said something about how she liked my hair. I told her it was the most expensive cut of my life. Then I told her about chemo and how the hardest part of losing my hair was my eyelashes and eyebrows. I told her I felt like I had been erased.

"The woman looked at me and said she could see eyelashes. I was ecstatic! I looked in the mirror and sure enough there they were. I felt so glamorous just knowing they were on their way back. My eyelashes and I *waltzed* out of that bathroom."

Recovering from chemo is really a "both/and" situation. You both celebrate your returning health *and* you grieve your losses. So you may get your taste buds, hair, and fingernails back. But maybe you've lost some body parts and now have hot flashes and osteoporosis.

The losses aren't just physical. You may have lost your career, your confidence, or a relationship. For sure you've lost a certain naiveté, an innocence about your own life. For me it was as if the pendulum swung the other way, and not only did I know that bad things could happen to me, I started to *expect* it. I found myself wondering what was going to smite us next? Was Wes going to be hit by a car on his bike? Would our house burn down? Would a gang of root weevils take down my rhododendrons?

The Port Authority

I wanted some time to myself to look over what I had just crossed. In September the Hawaii Cancer Center in Honolulu called to ask if I would give a talk in March on death, dying, and spirituality. After cleaning my slobber off the phone, I said, "I'd love to."

A few days later the mail brought one of those offers for five nights and six days on Maui for a ridiculously low price. These offers are so obnoxious because you usually can never go on the dates specified. It's like holding out a piece of pizza to a starving man and saying, "You can have this if in the next six seconds you can tell me the square root of 8,427."

The number of people that can do that in their heads is the same number that could actually go to Hawaii on the dates offered. And who knew we could do square roots in our heads? I looked at the dates and realized it the same week I was speaking in Honolulu. "We can *do* this!" I said. So we made our reservations.

I was telling Lynie about this. "A week in Hawaii in March will be so great. Now, to make my dream come true, I need to find a house-sitting gig." Because what I really wanted was a big stretch of time to sort things out.

A week later Lynie called back and said, "My in-laws in Kailua need someone to house-sit for them in March. They'll be going to New Zealand for two weeks. And they need someone to take care of Puna."

A house-sitting gig *and* a dog? In the meantime, Wes was invited to speak at a conference in Tokyo. This meant he would be staying only one night with me in the house in Kailua. So I would be *all by myself* in a house on the beach with a dog for two weeks. I was ecstatic.

I did not exactly pray for this. But I did put it out there to the Universe. The Universe/Mr. Martha Miyagi responded. It was a mystery, and I was content with that. Of course if we were going to be cavorting in swimsuits, then I really wanted to get my port out.

I scheduled the port removal a couple weeks before we left. So there I was lying on the table with Wes standing next to me, my port site filled with three gallons of local anesthetic. Gowned, gloved, and scalpel in hand, Our Friend The Surgeon paused before slicing me open and asked, "So are you and Wes going to do anything fun after this?"

"We're going to Hawaii!" I said grabbing his arm. His perfectly sterile arm. The moment I touched him I realized my mistake. I snatched my hand away hoping no one noticed but already everyone was groaning.

"Well, I guess we're doing this again," Our Friend said taking off his gown. I was so mortified, so embarrassed that it triggered the mother of all hot flashes. I fanned my neck, which oddly enough is attached to my chest, which is where my port was.

"Stop! That's sterile!" he shouted. "Somebody hold her arms down!"

Wes and the nurse grabbed my arms, and by then I was having an atomic hot flash. I could feel the paper beneath me getting soggy with sweat. Perspiration was running down my face and into my ears.

And I prayed, "Oh, God, take me now!"

No, Cockroach, you must endure.

I thought, "Okay, maybe this is the price of going to Hawaii." Perhaps I needed to learn to control my enthusiasm. Whatever it was, I felt like an idiot. But I was to have the last laugh that day. Just as Our Friend was pulling out the port, I said, "I want to save the port!"

"What? You want to keep it? What will you do with it?"

He was holding it up, all bloody with bits of tissue sticking to it. I looked at it and said, "I think I'll boil it and make soup!"

He screwed up his face. "E-e-w-w, that's so disgusting! Geez."

Victory! I had grossed out a surgeon! It was a big moment for me.

Plenty Papayas

Maui has always been a special place for me. My mother was born there in Lahaina, and my grandfather worked in the pineapple and sugarcane fields. My sister and I have vacationed there. I learned to snorkel there. It was to become even more special because it was on Maui that my new boob made its swimsuit debut.

When it came to breasts, I became like a teenage boy. I saw breasts everywhere and noticed their size and shape. I hoped I would get over this. The beach on Maui was a regular breast bonanza and I couldn't help pointing them out to Wes.

I never made any kind of judgment call, but just said under my breath, "Breasts."

He responded, "Time bombs." And that was the end of it.

I saw all sizes of breasts, some real and some unreal.

Here's the thing about breast implants: If you see breasts that look perfectly round like cantaloupes, chances are they are implants. I had one breast that was perfectly round and the other that was not. So here's what happened when I walked out on the beach in my swimsuit: nothing.

Nothing had ever happened before.

We stayed at an incredibly fancy hotel for dirt cheap. What we failed to notice in our vacation package was that we were required to listen to an agent give a talk about buying a condo. We innocently sat down at our "orientation" where a nice girl in an aloha-print uniform told us about the pools and the yoga classes and the restaurants. Then she said, "Now, what time would you like to schedule your presentation and tour?"

Wes and I looked at each other. "We don't want a presentation," he said.

She looked aghast. "Well, it's part of the package and it will take only a couple hours."

A couple of hours? Two hours doing something that I thought was stupid and uninteresting? When I could be snorkeling? I didn't come through cancer treatment for this. I started laughing.

"Oh, no," I said, "thanks, but I really can't take two hours out of my precious life for that." Wes and I grinned and stood up. "Good luck to you!" I said merrily and we headed to the beach.

Prayer is about losing yourself in the moment, joyful focus, and exhilarating concentration. Snorkeling is prayer. I think it's a miracle to be able to see underwater and breath at the same time. Unless there are whales or dolphins around, all you can hear is your breath. In-breath. Out-breath.

I love snorkeling along the coral reefs, where all the sea creatures hang out. But I don't mind being in the middle of the sea, just moving through the silky water facedown, sun reflecting on the sand below, and breathing in an expanse of blue. Or just floating and being gently rocked by the waves—an aquatic retreat of voluntary under-stimulation.

I've never been able to dive deeply while wearing a snorkel. For one thing, my ears hurt and for another, it's as if there is some invisible wall that keeps me from going down. But Wes is a master at it. So there we were swimming along and he was diving down and looking at things when he suddenly shot back up.

"There a gigantic sea turtle down there!" he said. I put my face down and sure enough, what I had thought was a big, flat rock was a turtle. Wes dove down to look at him, not getting too close. The turtle raised his head and looked up at me. A shiver of recognition went through me. We kept looking at one another, and the feeling I had was just like the one you get when you go to a twenty-five-year class reunion and you recognize someone, but you can't remember the person's name or if they were in your math class or homemaking or even if you liked them.

Then my mind got involved and said, "Don't be ridiculous. You can't know this turtle from somewhere." At that moment he put his head down.

Wes came back up and said, "I saw his face and he looks so wise."

"Yes. I think he was in my English class."

I thought about this all day. Could it be it was the Presence in me recognizing the Presence in the turtle? I sat with that for a long time and realized, yes, that was exactly it—a *namaste* experience.

Namaste is not just a yoga class sign-off like, "See you later, alligator!" The Hindi greeting *namaste*, means the Divine in me honors the Divine in you. I sometimes do it before I leave my desk to go see a patient. I place my hands together over my heart, close my eyes, and bow my head. It helps me to remember to turn down my mind and turn up my heart—listen for the voice of the Friend.

It was with this *namaste* awareness that I left Maui and flew to Honolulu to give the workshop "Mortality: Fact or Fiction?" I talked about death and dying. I told them about Addie Brown and her grandchildren. And I told them about one of my hospice patients, Cindy.

Cindy was twenty-one years old and had a brain tumor. She was an artist, which also meant she was a barista. For a while her boss and coworkers thought she was just a spacey artist because she mixed up the drinks and gave the wrong change. But then, after passing out one day, her doctors discovered she had a brain tumor.

They operated, but they couldn't get all the tumor, and at the time, there was no effective chemo. She had to move in with her mother because she could no longer work. She did pretty well for a while because she took steroids that kept her tumor in check. But it got to a point where even the massive doses of steroids were not working.

Fear of death was not an issue with her because she believed in reincarnation. The first time I met her she said, "I've died before. I used to live on the Olympic Peninsula, and that is the death I remember. It was no big deal. I fell into a hole, and then I came out on this side."

Because of the steroids, she gained a lot weight and lost mobility on one side. She hated hobbling around her mom's apartment.

The last straw was when she got stuck in the bathtub and couldn't get out. At this point she weighed about 220 pounds. Her mom had to call 911 and as she said, "These cute guys had to heave my naked ass out of that tub." It was humiliating for her.

So she said, "Debra, I'm tired of this. I want to stop taking my meds, and I figure I'll be dead in six days."

And because I had promised to officiate at her funeral, I got out my calendar and said, "Well, okay, let's see. I'm going on vacation in two weeks."

I'd known her for six months now and we were pretty close, so we could talk like this. I said, "Don't stop your steroids until the fifteenth. That'll make you dead by Tuesday. We'll have your service on Friday, and then Wes and I will leave for vacation on Saturday."

She loved this plan. Her family agreed because they could see how miserable she was. I saw her a few days later, and she held out this list and said, "Is there anybody you want to put on the list? This is a list of people I'm supposed to talk to after I'm dead."

I looked at the list and there was John Lennon, John F. Kennedy, Cousin Karen, Elvis, and Uncle Stevie. I just answered, "No, that's okay. My dead friends come to me in my dreams when they have something to say."

And she said, "Oh, okay, I'll do that."

Everything went according to plan: She stopped her meds and died six days later. I officiated at her memorial, and then we left for our camping vacation in Glacier National Park. We found a beautiful campsite and set up our tent. The very first night Cindy came to me in a dream.

We were on a beach together and Cindy looked fabulous. She was a healthy weight and was wearing one of those multicolored broomstick skirts. And she danced and twirled and said, "Oh, Debra, it's great, it's just great. I'm fine." I was delighted to see her looking so well. Then she stopped twirling and looked at me and said, "And thank you for helping me."

I said, "Oh, thank you for thanking me, nobody ever thanks me." Even in the dream I realized that was an idiotic thing to say. You know, I was having some kind of visitation and it's all about *me.* Then she put her hands on my shoulders and said, "And I have a message for my mother."

And I thought, "Oh, no," because her mom could get really cranky at times. So Cindy said, "Tell my mother she needs to spend more time on her spiritual life." Of course I said, "Okay," because how could I turn down a dead person, especially one who looked so good?

I awoke at sunrise euphoric. I don't mean happy, I mean *euphoric* as if I'd been smoking some killer bud. Or so I've heard. And I felt that euphoria the entire day. It was extraordinary.

So of course when we got home I called her mom and gave her the message. And as I feared, she was very annoyed and said, "Well, why did she tell *you?* Why didn't she tell me herself?"

I realized I had gotten myself into a dysfunctional supernatural triangle. So I said, "Well, if she shows up again, I'll tell her to stop in on your dream."

It was because of this experience with Cindy that I knew it was possible for the dead to communicate. It was really more than just a dream because it was too vivid. I smelled the ocean, heard the waves crashing, and felt her hands gripping my shoulders.

As I told this story I could see lots of people nodding their heads. This was great because now we were coming to the small group sharing experience. People are often squirrelly about this because they don't know the other people in their group, they're shy, they have gas pains, whatever. Predictably there was a little grumbling going on around the room as I split them up into groups. A couple people left. It didn't bother me, because I have never seen this part of a workshop fail.

I explained the ground rules: Speak from the heart and listen from the heart. Treat everyone and their stories/beliefs with respect. We used the Way of Council, which means one person speaks at time, whoever is holding the talking stick. The beauty of this is it helps you listen because you are not busy crafting what you are going to say. And it's great for people who sometimes need a moment to find the right word, or pause to think. No one can jump in and take over.

We didn't have a talking stick. I had intended to gather shells on Maui, but shockingly there were none to be found. So we passed out Magic Markers. I thought that was pretty cool because it had "magic" in the name. So every group went through the questions in the final session of "The Existential Expedition."

(1) What do you believe happens when you die?
(2) Is death the worst thing that can happen? Why or why not?
(3) What to you is the worst kind of death? Why?
(4) If you had to die right now, how would you like to die?

I gave them forty-five minutes but stretched that to an hour. The room was buzzing. At one hour and fifteen minutes, I begged them to reconvene to talk about this experience. They loved it and were surprised that they loved it.

One man said, "My group wants to talk some more, so we are all going out to dinner tonight!"

"Ask your waiter how he wants to die," I said, "then be sure to leave him a big tip."

Again, it was people connecting in moments of vulnerability—talking about how they wanted to die. I think that is why cocktail parties or parties in general are often so unsatisfying. Everyone is busy being attractive and happy and funny. It's not impossible to really connect with someone at a party, but it's rare.

As I was gathering my notes, two nursing students came up to me.

"We want to know about burnout," one of them said. "How do we keep from getting burned out?"

"You won't be burned out if you understand there is a gift in this for you. It's a two-way street."

She misunderstood me and said, "Okay, so I go in and don't expect anything back."

"No, no! I'm saying the opposite! You go to work and expect to find a gift in every encounter. It could be from a patient, a family member or a co-worker. It's not their responsibility to give it; it's your responsibility to find it. You must be alert."

The nurses I have seen who get burned out are the ones who are the martyrs—"Oh, I give so much of myself to my job."

I used to have a supervisor in hospice, who when she heard stuff like that would say, "Well, it don't *martyr* to me."

The other nursing student said, "I wanted to ask you about dreams. I took care of a lady and then I had a nightmare about her."

"Was she dead?" I asked.

"Not when I had the dream. She died about two weeks ago."

She was asking this because I talked about Cindy coming to me in my dream. We were quiet for a moment and then she said, "She reminded me of my mom, who died of cancer."

Ah, yes. "Just be aware of your emotions," I said. "You don't have to say anything to your patient, but if you are aware that this person is bringing up strong emotions for you, you can sort it out later and won't have to process it in your dreams."

I was a big fan of "sorting things out," and now I was going to get two weeks alone to do it. Wes and I drove out to Lanikai where we found a rustic Hawaiian bungalow set right on the water. The house looked east and every morning I awoke to the sun rising over the Mokulua Islands. There were two fish ponds and a bird feeder for me to manage. And there was Puna.

Puna was a pure white Samoyed who required a morning walk, food once a day, and drops in her eyes. You may think a ferociously furry dog like that would be miserable in the tropics. But Puna radiated peace, love, and tranquility.

Wes left early the next morning for Japan, and Puna and I settled into our routine. This consisted of me waking up to the sunrise and saying, "Holy-Jesus-God-and-All-the-Saints!" I said this every morning because it was so outrageously beautiful and I love sunrise. I made coffee, prepared a papaya with a little lime juice, and cooked an over-easy egg. Then I sat eating and watching the ocean. That's all I did. I didn't read. I didn't write. I just ate, sipped my coffee, and watched. I was relaxed but alert. What would the Unseen One show me today?

After breakfast I took Puna out for her walk on the beach. We walked until there wasn't any more beach. Walking with Puna was how I imagined it would be like walking with a movie star. Everybody recognized her and came up and said hi, and petted her. Even if they didn't know her by name, she was so attractive, people were compelled to say something.

She is like a celebrity among dogs, too. As we walked down the beach, dogs barked at her and strained at their leashes trying to get close to her. But she paid no attention to them. At first I thought, "Oh, my God, she is the Buddha—no dog fazes her." But then we were walking and there was one dog, a young beagle, with whom she was very interested in playing. So I stopped and they romped around for a while. This happened every day. If the beagle wasn't there, she chose some other dog.

I thought, "Hmm, she is very selective. Not every barking dog gets her attention. What does that mean for me?" And with absolute clarity I realized I didn't have to say yes to every project, but like Puna, choose only the ones that really captivate me.

I had to fly all the way to Hawaii to get that? Well, yes. I can't tell you why I didn't get it before, but I got it in a very deep way then. Part of it was having cancer—it really makes you see you haven't a moment to waste. The other part was that I was away and alone. There was no one needing me to be a certain way. I wasn't even asking anything of myself except to be alert and awake.

The weather cooperated in my quest to simply be. It rained. And rained. It was record-breaking rain, although it was usually dry first thing in the morning when Puna and I went for our walk. It wasn't just rain, it was torrential, non-stop rain with thunder and lightning. Buildings flooded, sewage pipes burst, the island of Oahu was a disaster area. Kailua beach had sewage in the water. This meant I had no guilt about not kayaking, swimming, snorkeling, or hiking. Roads were washed away. I couldn't go anywhere. Pure bliss.

The day I left the sun came out. I took my last walk with Puna. Then I gathered all my clothes, which were raggedy summer clothes, and dropped them off at a clothing bank. I wanted to leave my old self behind. And by that I mean the self that played with every dog who walked by.

Ten

RIB, RIB, HOORAY!

Dear Family, Friends, and Colleagues,

Today is my one-year anniversary of finishing chemo. Over the past year I've gotten used to my role as "the chaplain who had cancer treatment." So in addition to prayers, absolution, baptisms, Communion (real wine!), reflective listening, and sharing Divine wisdom, I now dole out advice on mastectomy camisoles (pockets for your drains!) and the importance of having a lightweight cotton knit warm-up suit that can double as pajamas and as day wear.

In my last update I said if tamoxifen didn't work out for me, I'd do my best to turn it into a cleaning product. I'm happy to say "Tamoxiclean" is now in Phase II trials. Something was causing a burning sensation in my mouth twenty-four/seven and no one in my cancer posse could figure it out. Was it the Zometa I received for my osteoporosis? The tamoxifen?

I went off the tamoxifen for five wonderful months. The hot flashes are now better, but my mouth is still an inferno. Because I have osteoporosis, I'm now taking raloxifene (or "relax the fiend" as we call it). It not only will prevent a recurrence, it will also build back my bones.

I'll admit it's been difficult at times to accept my body, which has been changed by surgery and chemopause. I think as we age we slowly and gradually revise our self-image. A few more gray hairs, a growing paunch, no big deal. But some events insist on a rapid revision—pregnancy is one of them, cancer is another.

I can't tell you how shocked I was to realize I could no longer do a decent cartwheel or fit into my high school blue jeans. It seems my fat cells, which for years have been localized in my thighs, have metastasized to the rest of my body. And where I used to pop out of bed like bread from a hyperactive toaster, I now ooze and groan my way to an upright position.

Nevertheless, in late August I felt that at last I was getting my health back. Some colleagues and I were talking about running the Seattle Half Marathon. I was lifting weights again. I took a week-long intensive yoga class. It was then that I went to Mazama in Eastern Washington to officiate at the wedding of some friends.

There I took my maiden voyage on a mountain bike. We were at the end of a two-hour ride during which I was smiling through clenched teeth and yelling, "Yeah, I love it, too! Yeah, feels so free!" I remember looking down at the big white marbles on my handlebars and realizing they were my knuckles.

We were two miles away from our starting point, going downhill on a rocky path. I was thinking, "I'm going too fast and feel out of control." The next thing I know I am writhing on the ground with the bike on top of me. My first thought: "Oh, %&$*!" All that chemo and surgery, and now I'm going to die in the dirt like a dog. (Even in my state of unbearable pain, I was pleased with that alliteration.)

Wes, realizing I was no longer behind him, came tearing back. He asked me all sorts of questions, but I couldn't speak. I could only move my fingers and toes to show him I did not have a spinal cord injury. He then noticed my arm, which was scraped and bloody and filled with dirt. Ever the infectious disease doc, he announced, "We must clean out that wound!" He proceeded to squirt his water bottle all over me.

Through clenched teeth I managed to croak out, "Least . . . of my . . . problems." He wanted me to get up because I was lying in the dirt in the broiling hot sun, but I simply could not get up. So he stood over me to provide shade. He is six foot three and was wearing a bike helmet and big, bulgy goggles. I looked up and felt as if I were going to be devoured by a giant insect— I welcomed it.

That was, in every way, the lowest point of this experience. I knew I had done something really bad to myself, and there was no going back.

Fast forward to the emergency room whose motto is, "We teach you how to wait." I was doing Lamaze breathing to deal with my pain. Finally, they took me back, took X-rays, and gave me an ultrasound. The nurse said, "We just had an acute M.I. come in," which is nationwide code for, "The attending physician is having a meal." Time became geologic, and just as we were entering the Jurassic period, the attending physician showed up.

He was very sweet, took my hand, and said, "First of all, I'm so sorry you had to come here tonight." I'm thinking, "Pain-pain-pain-pain-pain-pain-pain." Then he said, "Thank you for wearing your helmet." I'm still thinking, "Pain-pain-pain-pain-pain-pain-pain." Finally he said, "You have two broken ribs, but no internal injuries." He handed me a bottle of pain meds and said, "I don't want you to get pneumonia, so take these pills and ten deep breaths an hour."

Why didn't he just hand me a pair of steak knives and say, "Stick these in your eyes ten times an hour?" Pain-pain-pain-pain-pain-pain-pain.

So I missed two weeks of work, and I can honestly say this is the most pain I've ever experienced in my life—made my mastectomy look like a manicure. The two weeks I was home I spent eating, taking narcotics, and sleeping. I didn't catch up on projects, clean the house, or do anything interesting. Well—there was that first day I spent vomiting up narcotics and then vomiting from pain. That was pretty interesting.

I couldn't believe I was in so much pain for so long. Two broken ribs, and I was on narcotics for five weeks! Or was I becoming a drug addict? Nah—the constipation isn't worth it. Worst of all, the broken ribs never even showed up on the X-ray. Maybe they weren't really broken.

I saw my oncologist two months after the crash and was still wincing when I took a deep breath. The thing is, once you have cancer, what was formerly nothing could now be something.

"Broke two ribs because you fell off a bike?" she asked suspiciously. I tried to explain that I didn't simply fall, I crash-landed onto a ledge of rock. She still ordered a bone scan. This is exactly the kind of oncologist that I like, very thorough, leaving nothing to chance. I must admit it did cause my stomach to drop into my shoes when I saw her write, "Rule out mets" on the order. I knew she didn't mean the New York baseball team.

When the bone scan was over the tech got very excited. "Hey! I thought you said you had two broken ribs. I see six ribs and two fractures on each rib!" He sounded as if he had just won the grand prize at an Easter egg hunt. Sure enough, on the scan my rib cage looked like it was strung with Christmas lights. Very festive.

I did not consider this bad news. I felt vindicated. I wasn't such a baby after all!

Since I've been off chemo for a year, this will be my last update. I'm sure you are all breathing sighs of relief because you were afraid I'd start sending hernia, hemorrhoid, and Pap smear reports.

So thanks for caring and reading and responding to these updates. I'd like to thank my director and the Academy, but the orchestra is playing me off the stage, and my false eyelashes are coming loose from all the tears. And speaking of false, the boning in this strapless gown is poking my implant.

Love and Hugs,
Debra

Beginnings and Endings

I completed my first year of being off chemo, and there were all kinds of beginnings and endings happening around me. I had been following Lisa for four years. She had completed the last possible treatment for her cancer. We were now giving her palliative care: packed red blood cells, platelets, hydration. We referred to this as the "red wine, white wine, water" regimen. She already had hospice come in and do an initial assessment with her. She cut off her long hair before it all fell out and had a wig made that looked perfectly natural—until now. She had lost so much weight it perched on her head like a little blond nest.

If it had been any other patient in this situation, I would never have mentioned I was coming up on my chemo anniversary. But I had known Lisa for years and knew she would celebrate with me.

I knocked and slid open the door to her room. I was surprised to see she was fast asleep and even more surprised to see she was not wearing her wig. A soft knitted cap covered her head. I was just backing out her room when she opened one of her eyes, lifted her hand, and gave me a little smile.

"Come in," she said softly. "I have a question for you."

I gelled my hands. That was our policy at the clinic: "Gel in, gel out." It was like rubbing clean-smelling slime on your hands. Or blowing your nose without a tissue. Or shaking hands with a slug. You get the picture.

Lisa and I always joked about this because everyone who stands there rubbing his or her hands together looks like some mad scientist eager to inflict some horrendous pain. The unfortunate thing about this is we both thought that at times, it was true.

So I rubbed my hands together and said in my best Transylvanian accent, "Yes, my darling. What is your question before I stick the electrodes on your eyeballs?"

"The hospice nurses come in every couple of days. But at the end, don't you think they should be there all time, because what if I fall out of bed?"

I kept rubbing my hands together way after the gel had evaporated. I grabbed a rolling stool from the corner of the room and sat down. Then I lowered the seat and cleared my throat. I bought myself about fifteen seconds doing all of this.

"You won't fall out of bed at the end," I said.

"How do you know?"

"You won't have enough energy. You barely have enough energy to go to the bathroom now, right?"

"Right."

"Well, at the end, most people don't have a lot of energy and they usually go into a coma. If you're in a coma, you're not jumping around and you won't fall out of bed."

"Okay."

I rolled up close to the bed and took her hand. "If you're really afraid of that, you can have someone stay in the room with you." She didn't say anything for a long time, just lay there gripping my hand. I saw she was getting the "white wine" today.

Finally she said, "I told my daughter that Mommy is probably going to die from the cancer."

"What did she say?"

"She said, 'I don't want you to die, Mommy. What if I have a problem and need to ask you a question?' I told her, 'When you have a question, all you have to do is get very, very quiet and very, very still and ask your question. Then being as still and as quiet as you can, listen very carefully, and Mommy and God will give you an answer. And as you get older, when you are very quiet and very still, you will hear your own voice.'"

Here it was December and I had seen parents feverishly shopping and buying their children all kinds of toys and games and books and clothes. How many parents had thought of giving their children the gift of learning how to listen to God and listen to their own voice? Because I was fighting back tears, my voice was sort of thick when I said, "What an incredible gift you've given her."

"Thank you."

Get very still and get very quiet. I felt as if I spent most of my time as a chaplain telling people to check in with their breath, to quiet themselves, to listen. What if we all had learned to do this as children? Maybe I'd be out of a job.

There are times when I feel as if I am in the presence of some kind of Higher Being. That afternoon with Lisa I felt like that. She was thoughtful and filled with peace. I know some people who work with energy say that energy is just energy. Period. But I disagree. I've been with people whose energy felt scattered or chaotic or nervous. Maybe it's a matter of semantics. But Lisa's energy felt divine, and I wanted to sit there and bask in it.

Then she said, "It's wonderful to sit in the silence with you."

It's wonderful to sit in the silence with you. The words wrapped around me in that way I recognized as Spirit speaking. We sat for quite a long time holding hands in the silence, and I didn't tell her about my chemo anniversary.

Chemo Forever

There are three kinds of chemotherapy patients: (1) those, like me, who begin chemo and finish it; (2) those who have had chemo, have a recurrence, and are now on chemo again; and (3) those who never get off chemo.

Of course those of us in category 1 hope and pray we will never be put into categories 2 or 3. I've seen patients in all three categories. You might think the ones who are the most freaked are those who have a recurrence. Some people with a recurrence say at least they have a better idea of what to expect, because they know the routine. Other people feel they are going into a serious battle for their lives.

Getting a recurrence is like the scene in *The Shining* where Jack Nicholson hacks through the door with an axe and says in that evil voice, "Here's Johnny!" Except when you get a recurrence it's, "Here's cancer!" Again.

If you do get a recurrence, you hope you'll get chemo and finish it, just like with your initial diagnosis. But that doesn't always happen. Which brings me to category 3, never getting off chemo.

I have met many patients in this category who have come to a tentative peace about this. I say "tentative" because many people have told me every once in a while they will get all in a twirl about the fact that they are never getting off chemo. Chemo has failed to cure them. So total eradication being impossible, the idea is to keep the cancer from taking over. They think of their cancer as a chronic illness, like diabetes, something that will always have to be treated, because without treatment they will die sooner.

One of the problems with being in this category is that people don't know how to respond to someone on permanent or maintenance chemo.

My friend Stephanie says this happens to her all the time. "People will say, 'You look great! Are you done with chemo?' And I'll say, 'Oh, no, I'm never getting off chemo.' They look just stricken!" she said.

"They don't realize that my head is not in the same place it was with the very first big-slam-kill-it-all chemo. This maintenance chemo is in the background of my life. It's hard for some people to get that and they feel guilty that they haven't called or brought food. I have to explain that I don't need support in the same way now. Then there is this horrible awkwardness and they struggle to change the subject."

My guess is that their thoughts go something like this: "*Never* off chemo? Does that mean they haven't gotten rid of your cancer? If you go off chemo will you *die*?" The answers are yes, yes, and yes. It's this last part about death that really freaks people out.

I was in the clinic when the sister of a permanent chemo patient said to me, "I know this is keeping my brother alive, but I just can't believe that I'm looking at someone who is actually going to die."

I broke it to her gently that *everyone* she looks at is going to die. She left for the cafeteria in a state of shock.

If only we could get a little bit comfortable thinking about death. Death is *supposed* to happen.

What if no one wanted to leave a restaurant after the meal? The manager would come out and say, "You come, you eat, you leave. This is what you're supposed to do."

The problem is that we want to leave only after we've had the cocktail, appetizer, entrée, wine, salad, cheese course, dessert, coffee, after-dinner drinks, and a breath mint. It's sad but true that some people never make it to dessert or even to the entrée. That totally sucks. But nobody can *stay* in the restaurant forever.

We all want death to come when we are ninety-nine years old and fast asleep. I'm not saying we shouldn't grieve or that death is no big deal. But most people I meet can't even think about death and certainly don't want to talk about it. That's why the idea of never getting off chemo can be so mind blowing—it means death is just around the corner.

Most people in this category have a strong hope that some new experimental drug in the pipeline will save them. This is not an unrealistic hope. I saw this happen with AIDS and the multi-drug cocktails that yanked people from the grave. Because of newly discovered drugs, I've seen women who have inflammatory breast cancer live for years instead of months. So it is not crazy to hope for a miracle therapy—it's crazy not to.

So what *do* you say to someone who is on long-term chemo? "How are you doing with that?" or "How is this different from your other chemo?" or "Oh, wow. What do you do when you want to take vacation?" Force yourself to stay with it until the person on chemo changes the subject or until there is a 6.0 earthquake where you both are standing.

Some people with cancer never get back anything resembling their old lives. Sometimes the most they get is just life. Period.

This was the case with Elizabeth. She was twenty-four and had a one-month-old baby and a three-year-old at the time of her diagnosis. I met her at a cancer retreat I was facilitating four years ago. She's never been off chemo for more than a couple of months.

Knowing Elizabeth was like witnessing a bizarre drawn out version of the Stations of the Cross. Condemned to death at age twenty-five with Stage IV breast cancer.

"But we'll give you the best treatment we have," her doctors said. Now *there's* a cross to bear. She was not one of those women who sailed through chemo. She didn't have nausea, she had *severe* nausea—and exhaustion and diarrhea. The shots she gave herself to bring her white blood cell count up didn't give her "moderate" pain, they gave her severe pain.

I hadn't heard from her in a while, and out of the blue I received an e-mail. She wrote it at 3 a.m. Even after taking two sleeping pills, she was wide awake.

> I'm just struggling. I seem to know somewhere in the recesses of my brain that the only path to peace is through the Higher Power, but I'm stuck from there on out.
>
> I am obsessed with dying. Not afraid of it, really, just obsessed. How are my kids going to fare? My husband?

Who will make sure the turtle gets fed? Who will pop the pimples on Larry's back? What will I wear to be buried in? It goes on and on. It starts the first thing when I wake up in the morning and rarely lets up.

My disease is relatively stable, but I still have cancer in my liver and lungs. The ballpark guess for my prognosis is one to two years. So it's not like death is imminent for me yet, but it's still a lot sooner than I can be comfortable with, and I just can't stop thinking about it.

I got an e-mail update from the sister of my friend Tina, who passed away last May. Her sister wrote about the sense of peace everyone's feeling now that Tina is gone and how the last two years of Tina's life brought so much pain and anger, it was a relief to be past that.

It wasn't insensitively written at all. I understood completely what she was saying. It just makes me want to give that peace to *my* loved ones. I'm not suicidal or anything like that. But thinking that after the grief fades, my loved ones will be able to move forward, find joy again, while we are all now just riding this damned roller coaster like prisoners of war.

I guess I'm feeling tempted to give up. I know it's not time yet. I know I can't. The rational part of me knows all of this. But the pain and suffering this is causing everyone in my life, including myself, is just about unbearable right this minute, and knowing that there is peace waiting in the wings for all of us involved sounds a little tempting.

There is a lot of good in my life, too. But the good stuff is just as intense as the bad stuff. So mix it all up and you've just got a whole lot of intensity from every point in the spectrum, and it has coagulated to create this volatile bomb just about ready to go off in my head!

The next day I made myself a cup of tea and called her. She went over everything in the e-mail in more detail, speaking rapidly, barely taking a breath for over a half hour. You don't try to stop Niagara Falls; you stand in awe of it. But unlike the falls, I knew that when she was ready, Elizabeth would stop. Sometimes you just have to listen until someone is all talked out.

Her energy seemed so scattered, so I told her about listening for her breath as a way of pulling her energy back, a way of collecting herself.

"I know, I know," she said. "I should meditate. But I just don't see how anyone with small children can meditate."

Everyone has the picture of meditation as sitting for a half hour in the Lotus position. What if you can just take a mindful breath here and a mindful breath there? Doesn't this all add up?

I like to think of these mindful moments like calories. You can eat two thousand calories in one meal or you can eat small meals all day long. Either way, you end up with two thousand calories. You have one hundred mindful moments that last approximately fifteen seconds, and what does that add up to? About a half hour.

Anyone who meditates will tell you that very often, out of thirty minutes, exactly two minutes are spent being completely present. So I figure mindful moments are better than nothing.

"Elizabeth," I said. "I don't know how mothers with small children even manage to have a bowel movement, let alone meditate. So think of checking in with your breath as a kind of meditation for mothers you can do at any time."

"I certainly spend a lot of time in the bathroom these days."

"Perfect. This is a great place to check in with your breath—although I wouldn't advise *deep* breathing.

She laughed for the first time in thirty minutes. Humor can be a way of avoiding pain, but other times, it is grounding and brings you into the present.

"I try so hard," she said, "I really do."

"You have my permission to stop trying so hard. What if you just feel your feelings and don't resist?"

"That's it! I resist, I'm resisting, yes, that's it, because I don't like what is happening. But it is what it is, it's my journey. I'm in a support group that is really good because it is comprised of people who really get it, meaning they have cancer. But here's the problem with the people: they die. Two people last week told us they had just enrolled in a hospice program and I think, when is that going to happen to me? When am I going to die?"

The falls had started again. I listened and sipped my tea.

"Then there is my Mormon family who can barely speak to me now because I've taken my name off the roll. I've renounced my faith and my mother says, 'When you die you will go to Outer Darkness.' That's what they call it, Outer Darkness. So I don't talk with her much, and that leaves my friends out here in the sticks who are basically all fundamentalist Christians who love me but say they feel really bad I am going to Hell because I'm not saved.

"So many people feel bad because of me. And maybe it would be better if I *did* die soon so they can get on with their lives. But I'm twenty-nine years old, and this isn't how I thought my life would be. If I didn't have cancer I could finish school and be a productive member of society or at least help with the finances so the burden wouldn't be on Larry."

She stopped and I waited a while. Sometimes you have to give people a little space to take a breath, finish a thought, swallow. Then she said quietly, "I know it's a lot."

It was a lot but not the biggest anxiety assortment I'd ever encountered. "So let's start with you wondering when you're going to die," I said. "When you're waiting to die you're full of all kinds of expectations, you are in the future, and you're missing what is in front of you at this moment. What if you just lived your life?"

"Okay," she said softly. "But what about the people who think I'm going to Hell?"

"I have friends like that, too," I said. "Fundamentalist Christians are of my same faith, and it totally ticks me off. So I pretend they are believers of some very obscure religion of which I am very respectful. If they tell me I am going to Hell, I think, how fascinating this religion is! Because when I think of them this way, I can accept them."

"That's what you think, but what do you *do*, Debra?"

"I love them just the way I'd want them to love me."

"Oh, gosh, of course."

"Now what's this about your family getting on with their lives? We have this idea that our lives are on a trajectory that excludes pain or death or grief. So we think a painful experience blocks that path. Your children's lives haven't stopped because you have cancer. It's not like Elizabeth-and-her-cancer is a big boulder in the middle of the road and everyone is waiting for you to die so they can move on. Everyone's life is going on. Tina's sister just wanted her own pain and grief over Tina's cancer to end. Yes, it was a relief when Tina died, but no one's life stopped. Their normal activities stopped, what they wanted to do stopped, but their lives didn't stop. That *was* their lives."

I paused for a moment to let that sink in. I had to think about it myself, how we have this notion of life moving forward in a linear way, and we think it's only moving forward if we're doing what we want to do, and we don't experience any pain.

You never hear anyone say, "Well, I'm glad that beautiful cruise to Puerto Vallarta is over so now I can get on with my life."

Before we hung up she said, "You know, I'd like to shadow you some day."

"Oh, no. You'd be so disillusioned. Personally, I don't know how Jesus could stand having all those disciples around day and night. Not a moment to pass a little gas or pick his nose."

You don't know the half of it.

Like a Virgin

Chemotherapy proved to me (as if I didn't know it already) that love is not about sex. How could it be that Wes and I felt more love for one another than ever and were having less sex than ever?

First, there's the mastectomy, and there is no way you want to fool around while you are healing. I think I can safely say most men don't find Jackson-Pratt drains particularly appealing.

Then there is the chemotherapy that makes you feel like a piece of human fungus, and chemopause makes your vagina feel as if it's been sitting out on the Mojave desert for a few years. Add to that total loss of libido and physical sensation. All this makes for one wild, lusty night of reading in bed. Or watching videos.

I tried to think lustful thoughts, but I just found it exhausting. It wasn't like we didn't try, and this is when I discovered I was once again a virgin. If you're a woman and you think about your first sexual experience, you may remember it wasn't all that comfortable. I thanked God it was dark, and Wes couldn't see me grimacing.

I tried the Estring, which is a rubber ring that fits up into your vagina and gives your tissues a little hit of estrogen. I imagined it like some kind of evil drug dealer who doled out just enough estrogen to keep my tissues begging for more. I think it did juice things up a bit. The problem was I'm a small woman and with that ring taking up all that space, there wasn't room for anything else, if you get my drift. It's like parking a Humvee in a one-car garage and then trying to drive in a Volkswagen bus. As my oncologist said, "One size fits most."

We tried drowning ourselves in gallons of lubricant. The experience was still one of trying to thread a hot dog through the eye of a needle.

"Houston, we need to abort the docking procedure," I said one night.

"Roger on that," Wes said.

At least we kept our sense of humor.

Other patients have talked to me about this, too. Heidi said she felt her clitoris was about as sensitive as her knee. "I finally had to tell my husband to stop touching me down there," she said. "He couldn't believe it because we had a great sex life. I told him, 'It's not you. It's just that no one is home down there!'"

Wes and I had a great sex life, too, and I missed it. But I was still, as Wes put it, "intensely desirous of cuddling." That was true. I needed to be comforted about the fact that I wasn't interested in sex.

I consulted my naturopath. "The only thing I can think of," she said, "is a dildo to stretch out the tissues." She started to write it down on my chart and then paused. "I don't even know how to spell it."

My primary care physician nodded sympathetically when I told her the problem. "Okay, what you might try is some kind of—dilator."

"You mean a dildo," I said.

"Uh, yeah. You may have to start small and work your way up." She gave me the name of a sex-toy shop on Capitol Hill: Toys in Babeland.

Oh. My. God.

Yes?

I wore sunglasses on the way over and fully intended to keep them on while I was inside. But in my mind, there is no other way to do this kind of thing except directly.

"May I help you?" She was a sweet twenty-something girl with pierced eyebrows.

"Yes. I was on chemo and we didn't have sex for a while and I have no estrogen and my vagina has shrunk to the size of a drinking straw and I need something to get it back in shape."

"Yes, of course," said Pierced Girl.

Of course? Did she hear this all the time?

She took me over to three shelves of dildos. "These are silicone, these are latex, and these are blown glass," she said pointing to the different shelves. I know she said something after that, but I didn't get it because my mind was screaming, "Glass?! Isn't that dangerous? Why don't you just use plutonium?"

"You can't use silicone lubricant with silicone. You can only use water based or glycerine, although we don't recommend lubricants with glycerine because they can cause yeast infections. Now with latex toys you can use silicone lubricant."

I should be taking notes! Yeast infections? That's all I need.

I looked at the vast assortment of penises. They were like puppies at the pound. All of them seemed to say, "Pick me! Pick me!"

"How do I know which size to get?" I asked coolly. Never mind the fact that this whole venture had brought on a marathon hot flash.

"It depends on how many fingers you can get in your vagina."

"Oh, yes." I looked down at my hands and pondered this question. Did she include the little finger? Because that's a *lot* smaller than the other three. That could throw off the entire calculation.

"I'll let you make your choice and just let me know if you need any help."

"Thank you so much." You would have thought I was buying gloves at Macy's. I quickly ruled out the glass and latex varieties. But the dildo buffet was still overwhelming, so I ruled out anything that looked real because I had the real thing at home.

Then I remembered what my doctor said about starting small. There were three that were exactly alike, except they were small, medium, and large. Perfect. I picked up the small one: thirty dollars! Forty for the medium and forty-five for the large. I wasn't about to spend one hundred and fifteen dollars on dildos! Once I graduated to the large, what would I do with the small and medium ones? Donate them to the church rummage sale?

I would just have to start big. I grabbed Papa Bear off the shelf and waved at Pierced Girl. "I'll take this one."

"Alright. I'll be right back." She returned with two sealed bags. "Purple or black?" she asked.

"Well, black does go with everything," I said, "but the purple's irresistible." I immediately named him Prince.

Now I had to get some fancy lubricant for Wes and me. Clearly our common drugstore stuff wasn't cutting it. There were testers for every brand. On every shelf was a box of tissues so you could wipe off your fingers. So thoughtful.

So I tried Maximus, O'My, Sliquid Silk, Babelube, Infinity, and Pink. Pink was in a handblown Italian glass bottle so you could leave it out on your nightstand and no one would walk in and scream, "Oh, my God! Lubricant!"

Instead they'd probably say, "Oh, what a beautiful bottle." Then they'd pick it up, and because it's slippery, drop it on your floor. Then you'd have lubricant everywhere and a lot of explaining to do. But what are they doing sniffing around in your bedroom?

Anyway, I ended up buying a bottle of "Gun Oil" because I liked the way it felt, and I knew Wes would find the name hilarious. Unlike Pink, I wouldn't keep it on the nightstand but perhaps in the garage.

I was feeling pretty wild now and decided to buy some erotic literature. I chose a book whose cover looked very cultured and sophisticated. It was a collection of stories. I'll tell you right now that the stories where they hop in the sack after knowing one another only ten minutes just didn't turn me on. I got anxious and started talking out loud saying things like, "You need to pay attention to your relationship first!" or "You both have communication issues." I was doing pre-marital counseling with erotica.

The stories that work for me are where they secretly love one another for ages, are afraid to admit it, finally confess, and *then* hop in the sack. So I read a story and then Prince and I would get to work, paving the way for the Real Thing. It really was work at first because there was a fair amount of discomfort. I looked upon it like dental hygiene, although I've never once had an orgasm while flossing—yet.

At night, while Wes read his science journal in bed, I read my erotic lit. After a story or two I would fling the book on the floor and say, "Honey, step away from that journal!"

Like my taste buds, gradually things came back. Lights were flickering in the house. I'm convinced there is no way to rush it. The best thing to do is pretend you really *are* a teenage virgin and you will only allow kissing. You might say, "I'm not one of those slutty cheerleader types!" and gently smack your partner. Then think about your parents coming home any minute. Then imagine all the girls at school finding out. Then all the boys. Then . . .

Well, it worked for us.

Son Stroke

Mr. Palmer had prostate cancer. I loved visiting him in spite of the fact that he was a Republican who fully supported the U.S. military in Iraq and thought it was wrong to be gay. He said it took him a while to get used to the idea of women ministers, but now he thought they were okay. As if to prove this, he never called me by my first name, but always called me "Reverend."

I tried to view him as perhaps Jesus viewed Zacchaeus, the hated tax collector. He was just a guy doing his job with the wrong opinions. He always insisted we pray together before I left. If his nurse was there, or anybody for that matter, he would grab their hands in his big meaty ones and make them pray with us.

Once we were talking about all the diseases that were referred to by their initials, like ADD and ADHD and SAD.

"I think it's all a bunch of hooey," he said. "Seasonal Affective Disorder! You know what that is? That's a bunch of cream puffs sitting around and being depressed about the weather. Snap out of it!"

"We do have more overcast days in Seattle than anywhere," I said. "I think some people really need more sunlight, maybe . . ."

"And all these kids with ADHD! Can't sit still in class so now they call it a disease. It's just being bratty, that's all it is. And the spineless teachers who can't control their students are probably these same cream puffs who have SAD. They probably . . ."

He stopped in the middle of his sentence and asked, "Do you have any children?"

"What?!"

I was used to this with Mr. Palmer. It was as if someone in his brain suddenly slammed on the brakes. His thoughts would screech to a halt, make a sudden turn, and then take off again.

He repeated his question. "Do you have any children?

"No."

"You should have children so you could love them."

Instead of telling him there was no way I could ever have children, I was able to demonstrate it because a sudden hot flash came upon me. I whipped out my fan, smiled at him, and began fanning myself.

"Oh," he said. "Well, you should have *had* children."

Wes and I loved kids but never wanted any of our own. Over the years we were constantly asked if we were going to have kids. We rarely came clean because saying, "We don't want children," was like saying, "We don't want world peace." Most people thought not wanting children was simply *wrong*. So usually I was silent and let people think we were "trying," although I knew this ploy wouldn't work forever. We stopped getting asked when I turned forty-five. Instead they started asking if we were thinking about adopting.

I cleared my throat and said to Mr. Palmer, "We had a dog."

"Ah, yes—a dog."

I tried to look a little sad, as if I had been hoping for a child, but I could tell he didn't buy it. "Oh, no," I thought, "Here it comes, the sermon on Why You Should Have Had Kids."

"I've had both children and dogs," he said quietly. He paused for a moment before saying, "And I will tell you something, Reverend." I braced myself. "Dogs are more loyal and much more fun!"

Then he burst out laughing. He was still chuckling and wiping his eyes when he said, "My son was the biggest pain in the ass I've ever had."

"But what about having children so I could love them?"

"Well, that was before I knew you had a dog."

We were both laughing like jackals when the nutritionist poked in her head. She looked puzzled and quickly said, "I'll come back later."

That just made us laugh harder. My conversations with patients were not entirely about spirituality any more than the nurse's conversations were entirely about the patient's health. I was not some mystical ATM where patients made spiritual transactions. I think the best of us chaplains offer a bit of friendship. Perhaps it is a brief and temporary one. It's a lot of listening, some counseling, a bit of self-disclosure, and sometimes a dash of affection. But the whole of the relationship is greater than the sum of its parts. Sometimes I felt the teeniest bit guilty because most of the time I have so much fun being a chaplain.

I must admit there were times when I wished like crazy someone would walk in just so they could see I was earning my paycheck. But no one seems to barge in when a patient is crying in my arms, or when we're praying, or on Ash Wednesday when I'm dispensing ashes.

Son Light

What Mr. Palmer didn't know was every two weeks I got to have an hour-long conversation with a young man who was just the right age to be my son. His name was Miles, and his mother, Eve, died of breast cancer the year before. She was a smart, beautiful, feisty woman who adored her son, even as she sometimes complained about his teenage attitude. She was divorced from his father, and although Miles lived with her most of the time, his parents had shared custody. I loved visiting with Eve because we would compare notes on different Buddhist books we had read. We also talked about death all the time.

Of course we had all these death talks while she was getting treated, and it looked like the chemo was working. Then, just like Kari, when it was clear the treatment was no longer working, she didn't want to talk about dying. She focused her attention on Miles and asked if I would just have a conversation with him. She was worried about him.

This all happened when I had that fabulous office. So we went in there and sat at the little round table and talked. We talked about his mom dying and how he felt about it. I remember him crying and looking at me and saying, "I don't think I've ever been as present as I am at this moment."

So when it became clear Eve was dying, that there was no more chemo left, she said to me, "Promise me you'll see Miles." I promised.

Eve died the day after her birthday, a week before school started. Miles wisely delayed entry to the university, and took the quarter off. He flew back East and visited his grandmother. Then he returned to Seattle, worked at Barnes and Noble, and lived with his dad and stepmom.

He started seeing me about four months after Eve died. At first I met him at Starbucks on my day off. He offered to pay me, but I refused. I think he felt bad about that so he started coming to see me every other week at the clinic. Because I didn't have an office, I would scrounge around for consult rooms on any floor I could find. I didn't mind this room hunt, or the "knock and peek," as Miles called it. It gave a sort of Joseph-and-Mary-looking-for-an-inn flavor to it all. It always felt like a small triumph to find a space.

We just talked like friends—sort of. I always steered the conversation around to talking about his mom. The first year after a death is one of the hardest. And Miles not only lost his mom, but his home and all his high school friends.

We talked about school, his girlfriend, and whether or not he would get a summer job. We discussed who were the Buddhas in our lives—those people who drove us crazy and made us see where we lacked compassion or love or understanding or patience. We talked about restaurants and we talked about God. Miles was proud of having had a bar mitzvah, but he never went to temple. I can safely say he considered himself "spiritual not religious."

He was refreshingly not self-absorbed unlike many eighteen-year-olds I've met. After he talked for a little while, he'd always turn to me and say, "So how are *you*?" Then I would tell him about what was going on with me. Once he brought me flowers as a thank-you and for our anniversary he made cookies. So I wasn't exactly a chaplain to him. I, for sure, wasn't a mom, not really like an aunt, and too old to be a sister. So I was his friend.

He had a tendency to intellectualize things, and because he was very smart, it was easy for him to do. So I often found myself saying, "Well, how do you, *you*, Miles feel about that?" Around every holiday, I asked, "What did you and your mom used to do on this holiday?"

I had asked a nurse if she thought my meeting with Miles was doing him any good. "Are you kidding?" she said, "A teenage boy who gets himself here every two weeks must be getting *something* out of it."

It turned out our regular meeting day was his mom's birthday, the next day being the one-year anniversary of her death. I wanted to give him something, a card, a book, what? Nothing seemed right. When he arrived that day I greeted him with a hug and the words, "Congratulations. You made it through the first year." He had gone through a whole year of holidays without his mom. "I'm buying you a drink," I said.

We walked over to the Thomas Building and we both got lattes and then sat on a bench at the water's edge.

"Do you think something happens physically to a person who witnesses a death?" he asked.

"Why?"

"It just feels like ever since Mom died, everything is more intense—everything is brighter, louder, softer, harder."

"I don't know for sure," I said, "but it wouldn't surprise me. But maybe it's that seeing your mom die makes you realize how beautiful life can be and how short it is. So now everything seems more alive."

We just sat there silently thinking about that. Then a guy in a raft came floating by. He had a long pole and jammed it into the water every so many feet. "Just seeing if it's deep enough to bring my boat in here," he said.

"He's plumbing the depths," I said. "Just like dating. Testing to see whether someone is deep enough for you to bring in your whole self."

Miles started laughing, "Yeah, yeah, exactly." Then he talked about his girlfriend and how their relationship was going. And as I sat there a feeling of pure bliss settled over me. Most of my friends who had kids Miles's age never had conversations like this with them. Miles could be my son, but if he were, would we be having this conversation? If I had my own kids, I probably wouldn't have the energy for Miles.

There must be some long German word that means a glimpse of the road not taken, seeing how sweet it could be, but at the same time feeling perfectly content with the choice you've made. It was as if Eve was sitting there with us too, saying to me, "Isn't it great? I wanted you to have this."

Now What?

So how will my life be different after cancer? Honestly? Not too much different. I've stopped going to things like the Turkish Gerbil Harmonica Concert just because the person who has invited us is nice. I keep more white space on my calendar.

I love myself with the extra ten pounds. The hair I lost came back gray, and it is now sticking up out of my head like little silver wires. I was cleaning out my basement, and in my trunk I found my high school cheerleading uniform (I was not one of the slutty ones), along with a ten-inch ponytail I had cut off when I was nineteen. It was perfectly virgin hair, not highlighted, bleached, or tinted. I showed it to my hairdresser who said, "That ponytail is *way* more valuable than your present hair." I tried not to be offended. So I sent off my high school ponytail to become a wig. I hope it's a big one.

Our sex life is better thanks to Prince and Gun Oil, although I did have one very bad experience. We were coming back from a vacation and I unconsciously, thoughtlessly, *stupidly* threw the Gun Oil into my carry-on luggage.

"Ma'am we need to check your bag," said the woman at the X-ray machine.

"Oh, yeah, sure. Is it my inhaler?" Sometimes my inhaler is mistaken for a small pistol. She dug through my bag and pulled out the bottle.

"Gun oil?" she asked loudly.

Everyone froze. I mean, *everyone*. Of course this triggered a hot flash. Little beads of sweat were forming on my forehead. Why didn't I just turn myself in as a terrorist?

A big, burly TSA guy came over. "Dump out your bag."

The woman was still examining the bottle. I leaned over and whispered, "It's lubricant." Our eyes met and there was a flicker of recognition, of empathy.

The burly man was just about to take the bottle from her when she snatched it away and said, "We have everything under control here."

I still had to dump my bag and let them paw through nasal decongestant, a half-eaten protein bar, a hairbrush that looked like a Shih-Tzu, and a package of facial oil-blotting papers. Humiliating?

This is a test of the Universal Humiliation System. If this were an actual humiliation you would feel worse. This is only embarrassing.

Besides the above example, I continue to hear the Spirit's voice in the most absurd circumstances: while getting a hair cut, cleaning the toilet, waiting at the checkstand, or peeling carrots.

I have stopped trying to please everyone. I took my lesson from Puna, and I am selective about where I'll put my energy.

I truly have let go of my desire to have my sister and parents reconcile. I mean, I would love it, but my happiness is not dependent upon it.

And then there's Max. Wes and I decided to write Max's owner and make one final plea and offer for the precious terrier. I hadn't let go of my desire for Max, but I had let go of the outcome. I walked to his house for the last time, notebook in hand to write down their house number so I could address the letter. I noticed no one was home, so I thought, "I'll play with Max one more time."

Just as we were finishing our usual game of fetch, his owner's wife drove up. She got out of her car. "Don't go!" she said. "I wanted to talk to you about Max." Busted! In spite of the forty-degree weather, I had a hot flash.

She approached me with a big smile. I realized I wasn't breathing. "So," she said brightly, "Are you still interested in taking Max?"

"Yes, y-yes."

She was most gracious as she explained that as a Korean, she did not share her American husband's attitude about dogs as pets. Although her husband loved Max, they realized he would have a better life with me and Wes.

I picked up Max the next day and took him straight to a groomer who cut off all his dirty, matted hair. He is such a joy to us—you would think he had been ours all five years of his life.

It took us two years to get Max, and we received him only after I really, *truly* let go. I am working this realization into other areas of my life.

I light a candle every morning to remind me that on this day, I will bring light to the world. Just this one day.

Amen.

ACKNOWLEDGMENTS

My deepest gratitude to Bill Bush, MD, who was the first guy to see my mammogram and say, "Hmmm." Without him I wouldn't be writing these acknowledgments.

Many thanks for the excellent care I received from Dave Byrd, MD; Frank Isik, MD; Hannah Linden, MD; Mary Migeon, MD; and Leanna Standish, ND. Thanks to Wesley C. Van Voorhis, MD, PhD, for answering all my infectious disease questions.

Deepest admiration and respect to all the nurses at the Seattle Cancer Care Alliance, particularly my chemo nurse Sherry Joseph, RN, who was always a calm presence and shining light. I'm grateful to Barb Jagels, RN, nurse manager, who said a swear word when I told her my diagnosis and encouraged me to write e-mail updates for the staff.

Thank you to everyone who received my e-mails and responded with, "You should write a book!" As you can see, I took your suggestions seriously, and I now encourage you to buy this book. Buy several copies.

To my boss, Rev. Dr. Stephen King, I can only wonder what you did in a previous life to have to put up with me in this one. You have been generous and understanding beyond belief. Thank you. I'm also grateful to my chaplain colleagues who covered for me after my surgery and supported me during and after treatment.

My sister Lyn Monahan and my parents Mary and Syd Jarvis know me quite well—and they still love me. Thank you for interrupting your lives and coming to Seattle to be with me. Your presence was healing.

Dad, thanks for telling me, "You can do anything if you put your mind to it." Mom, thanks for always saying, "Be yourself."

I really don't know how I could breathe without Carla Granat, Trudy James, and Lisa Brihagen in my life. Thank you for bringing food, giving rides, sending cards, and doing energy work on me. My heartfelt thanks to Carla who read every single word of this book and was wonderfully honest. Oh, and thanks for holding my hair back while I puked in the salad bowl after the mountain bike accident. To Wes, I must express my appreciation for putting up with my long, loud phone calls to the above-mentioned troika.

Stephanie Donich, who started Cool Headz Hats, has been an amazing friend to me. Thank you for your support and sharing your MiraLAX with me when I was taking all that oxycodone after the mountain bike crash.

A very special debt of gratitude is owed to Sara Sarasohn at National Public Radio, who accepted my first commentary and encouraged me to write more of them.

If it weren't for Sara, Gary Luke at Sasquatch Books would not have heard me on the air and contacted me about writing a book. Gary is a scream and a great editor. Gary, thanks for saying that you too felt there were "magic stars" around this book. Gary is surrounded by gorgeous women at Sasquatch Books. I'm not kidding. One who I know for a fact is gorgeous inside and out is Rachelle Longé, who has been an enthusiastic and insightful editor. Thanks also to Sarah Hanson, Tara Spicer, and the rest of the Sasquatchettes.

Deepest gratitude to Tess Gallagher, who built a fire under me that weekend and got the book really going way before Gary ever called me. I'm grateful for your love, friendship, guidance, and generosity. Your poetry feeds my soul.

Thank you, Joan De Claire for your proposition on the pre-position. You are a skilled writer and a wonderful friend.

I hold a special place in my heart for the folks at University Congregational United Church of Christ, where I am recognized as specialized minister and something of a nutcase. Your support of my ministry and me is deeply appreciated.

I'm grateful to our dog Max for his unconditional love. It may seem weird to thank him in print because I know he can't read—yet. He's *very* smart.

And finally, I express my humble gratitude to all patients, family members, and staff. You continue to teach me more than you will ever know.

ABOUT THE AUTHOR

Debra Jarvis is an ordained minister in the United Church of Christ. She has worked as a hospice spiritual counselor and currently serves as a general oncology chaplain for the Seattle Cancer Care Alliance. She is a commentator for National Public Radio and frequently speaks at conferences and workshops on cancer, death and dying, medical staff care, spirituality, and the importance of quality chocolate.

Jarvis received her Master's in Divinity from Northwest Theological Union, Seattle; an MA in Christian Arts from New College, Berkeley; and a BA in Communications from UC Berkeley. She is board certified through the Association for Professional Chaplains (APC) and is a Certified Thanatologist through the Association for Death Education and Counseling (ADEC).

Jarvis is the author of *The Journey Through AIDS: A Guide For Loved Ones and Caregivers* (Lion, 1992); *HIV Positive, Living With AIDS* (Lion, 1990); and *Take It Again—From The Top* (Lion, 1986). She wrote and directed the play *Don't Think About Monkeys*, which toured Washington State with support from the White Horse Foundation.

She lives in Seattle with her husband Wes Van Voorhis and Max, their mighty cairn terrier. Visit Jarvis's Web site at www. debrajarvis.com and her blog at www.itsnotaboutthehair.blogspot. com.

The author is donating a percentage of the proceeds from this book to the Healing Journeys "Cancer as a Turning Point" conference and to the Harmony Hill Retreat Center, which provides free conferences and retreats for cancer survivors, patients, loved ones, and caregivers.